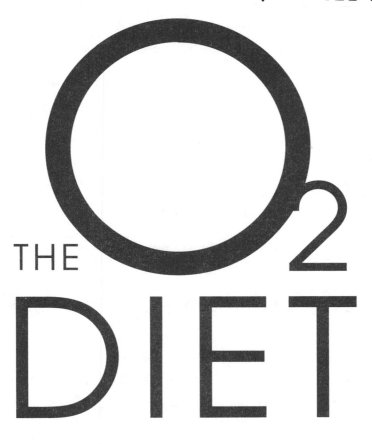

THE O₂ DIET

THE CUTTING EDGE
ANTIOXIDANT-BASED PROGRAM
THAT WILL MAKE YOU HEALTHY, THIN, AND BEAUTIFUL

KERI GLASSMAN, MS, RD, CDN
WITH SARAH MAHONEY

RODALE

© 2010, 2011 by Keri Glassman

First published in hardcover by Rodale Inc. in 2010

This paperback edition published in 2011

All rights reserved. No part of this publication may be reproduced or transmitted in any form or by any means, electronic or mechanical, including photocopying, recording, or any other information storage and retrieval system, without the written permission of the publisher.

Rodale books may be purchased for business or promotional use or for special sales. For information, please write to: Special Markets Department, Rodale Inc., 733 Third Avenue, New York, NY 10017.

Printed in the United States of America

Rodale Inc. makes every effort to use acid-free ⊗, recycled paper ☺.

Book design by Christopher Rhoads

The Library of Congress has cataloged the hardcover edition as follows:

Glassman, Keri.
    The O2 diet : the cutting edge antioxidant-based program that will make you healthy, thin, and beautiful / Keri Glassman.
        p.   cm.
    Includes bibliographical references and index.
    ISBN-13: 978–1–60529–518–3   hardcover
    ISBN-10: 1–60529–518–3   hardcover
    1. Reducing diets.   2. Antioxidants.   3. Nutrition.   4. Health.   I. Title.
    RM222.2.G5376 2009
    613.2'5—dc22   2009038289

        Paperback ISBN-13: 978–1–60529–167–3

Distributed to the trade by Macmillan

2   4   6   8   10   9   7   5   3   1   paperback

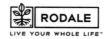

We inspire and enable people to improve their lives and the world around them

For more of our products visit rodalestore.com or call 800-848-4735

To the Roo and the Bean,
the O_2 of my life

Contents

The Science
of the O₂ Diet

Trans fats. White sugar. Aspartame. Sodium. Isn't it strange that we spend so much time talking about the many ways "bad" foods hurt us? We know how red meat raises our cholesterol and the ways pastries make us fat. But few people—even my most savvy clients—can explain how healthy foods truly help us.

Sure, you've read a lot about how eating well leads to greater health—everybody knows you are what you eat, right? But to you, isn't that some vague, abstract idea? In your mind, aren't you just saying, "Blueberries help my blah-blah"? Don't you think if you actually knew what those blueberries did for you, you'd be more motivated to order them for dessert? Once I get my clients eating delicious foods packed with nutrients, they still seem shocked at how these foods have the power to change them *right now*. Stunned, they'll say, "I have lost 12 pounds, but I can't believe how great my energy is, and everyone is commenting on my gorgeous skin!"

It's as if any benefit to eating well—beyond weight loss, that is—is a total mystery. But it shouldn't be that way. Of course, one of the right-here, right-now payoffs for eating great foods is shedding excess pounds, and these days, many people are right to be focused on that. But the other perks of eating good-for-you foods—glowing skin, more energy, a sharper mental focus—are just as predictable, just as immediate, and every bit as important. You deserve them in your life, too!

That's why I came up with the O₂ Diet. It's a satisfying 32-day plan that will help people get over that disconnect. If you can *feel* good and focus on enjoying healthy foods instead of focusing on the scale, your energy will be off the charts. Your skin will look great. You'll sleep soundly. Then you will want to continue to eat well, which means you'll continue to lose weight, keep it off for good, and enjoy your life along the way. I want to teach you that yes, you really are what you eat, and I'll show you how learning to love the right foods—not just avoiding the wrong ones—can reshape your health from the inside out. As you learn to use these foods to their full advantage, you'll be amazed at how powerful you will feel. With so much nutrition at your fingertips, you'll wonder why it took you so long to fall head over heels in love with healthy eating.

Eating nutrient-rich foods will perform minor miracles inside your body, from reducing the plaque in your arteries to preventing your brain from slowing down—you'll always remember to shave both legs! (Oops, am I giving too much away about my own multitasking overload?)

And there will be big exterior changes, too. Yes, you'll lose weight, and your love handles will disappear. But your skin will get softer and glow. The tiny lines in your face will be less noticeable. Your hair will shine, and your nails will be stronger than ever. Your partner will love the way your libido has perked up. You'll sleep better, relax more, and stress less.

In short, you'll be able to wake up every morning and love how you feel and like how you look. And the best part? It is simple! If you focus on the fact that you need to *eat more* of the right foods, you will be healthier. You will *feel better*. And you will *look great*.

The O₂ Diet includes a groundbreaking 32-day plan. Each day, you'll consume foods so jam-packed with nutrition that you'll get about 30,000 points of what experts call ORAC value. ORAC stands for oxygen radical absorbance capacity (yes, it's a mouthful!). It's a scale that measures how well the components of a food mop up the free radicals in the bloodstream. Eating about 30,000 ORAC points will boost the antioxidant power of your blood at least 10 to 25 percent.[1] This is one of those rare nutritional areas where more is better: For the first 4 days, you'll consume

50,000 ORAC points daily, then you'll take in 30,000 units daily for the remainder of the plan—almost all of them from some of the healthiest fruits and vegetables available.

With the O₂ Diet, you won't have to count calories, grams of fat, or fiber—I'll just ask you to keep track of ORAC points of certain healthy foods. Why? Because while researchers are still learning precisely how these foods work, they do know that foods high on the ORAC scale can help you lose weight, improve memory and cognition, prevent cancer, reverse heart disease, lower stress, and protect joints. They minimize your skin's lines and intensify its glow. What's more, just by learning to navigate among these very healthy foods—and feeling empowered by doing so—you'll end up at your healthy body weight. You'll be your smartest, most energetic, healthiest, and most beautiful you—inside and out!

Before you can dive into the O₂ Diet, eating the healthiest, most scrumptious foods on the planet, you need to understand exactly what these foods do. That way, you'll appreciate their power and grasp why it's to your best advantage to put as many of these healthy, natural compounds into your body as possible, every single day.

how antioxidants work

As much as I want to race right into the good stuff—explaining how much you can do for your health with yummy things like cherries, avocado, and even chocolate—we have to start with a quick chemistry lesson. (If we can get a little cerebral right now, the concepts will stick—and I promise the lesson will be over soon!)

The cells in our bodies are made up of molecules, and molecules are made up of atoms. When we're young, right through our teenage years, all those little bits and pieces renew themselves at a fast clip, and cell renewal is brisk. We're at our athletic peak. Our skin is plump and smooth. Even if we stay up all night or push ourselves in a hard workout, we shake off the aftereffects and bounce right back the next day. Remember when you could pull off an all-nighter, then spend the day at the beach, then still go dancing that night?

But as we begin to age—and I mean as early as our twenties—cells start breaking down faster. When a cell dies, it releases a lonely little oxygen molecule known as a free radical. These tiny homeless bits of oxygen are what cause so many health problems: They have been linked to premature aging (hello, crow's-feet!), heart disease, cancer, a host of other illnesses, poor immune function, and even Alzheimer's disease.

How can oxygen be bad? you're probably wondering. *Isn't oxygen good for us? Don't we need it to stay alive? After all, it's in the air we breathe and in the water we drink.* You're right—oxygen *is* absolutely essential. Oxygen equals life. But it has to be that beautifully balanced O_2 molecule. It's so important I'm naming this book after it!

How do single oxygen molecules (aka free radicals) cause so much mischief? Think of a free radical as a pinball careening around inside your body, constantly smashing into other cells, or think of it as somebody who keeps bombarding you with e-mail jokes you've seen 20 times. The free radical disrupts normal cell functioning—the cells can't do their jobs properly because this little guy keeps storming the gates. The fatty acids in our cell membranes are especially vulnerable to these assaults, as are the core components of DNA. We can see evidence of oxidative damage all around us: It's what causes metal to rust and what turns a newly sliced apple brown in a matter of hours.

What do brown apples and rusty nails have to do with crow's-feet? It's all the same oxidative process. A certain number of free radicals is absolutely normal. Even the healthiest people—living in the purest communities, eating a perfect organic diet, and meditating all their stress away—have free radicals piling up in their bodies. The reality is that aging is 100 percent natural and 100 percent inevitable.

In a perfect world, we'd all be well protected against oxidative damage. We would consume basic levels of antioxidants, including vitamins A, C, and E, as well as dozens of other phytonutrients found in common foods. We would be protected from sun and environmental damage, sleep restfully each night, and never stress. The antioxidant chemicals would enter the bloodstream and do a great job of eliminating free radicals.

In a nutshell, free radicals cause damage; antioxidants protect us from them. Here is an illustration that shows how antioxidants pair with free radicals to form a balanced O_2 molecule.

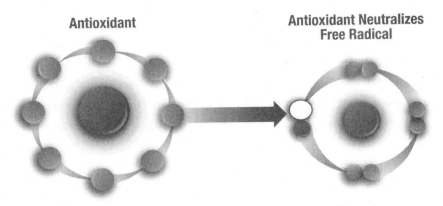

Antioxidant

Antioxidant Neutralizes Free Radical

You don't need to memorize dozens of long chemical names to follow the O_2 Diet. Just know that antioxidants work in many different ways. They can:

- "Quench" the single oxygen molecules by destroying them.
- Help the homeless oxygen molecules bind with other molecules in a less disruptive manner.
- Prevent the breakdown of the molecule in the first place, so that the free radical is never created.
- Encourage the body to crank out more of its own arsenal of antioxidants, such as lipoic acid.

In a perfect world, this process would happen on its own. The problem, though, is that few of us live in that world, and we have lots more than simple aging to worry about. We live in cities full of pollution, cigarette smoke, and radiation. We work stressful jobs that alter our bodies' chemistry for the worse, and then we deprive ourselves of the sleep that would heal us—if only we had the time. Some of us take medications to stay healthy, but they, too, can cause cells to break down.

As the free radicals build up in our bodies, the health consequences can become serious: These highly reactive cells have been linked to many illnesses, including heart disease—the number-one killer of men and women in America—a variety of cancers, dementia and other cognitive problems, poor eyesight, and even arthritis. Free radicals take a toll on us physically, causing skin to wrinkle and sag before it should. And perhaps the sneakiest effect of all is that too many free radicals means we just don't feel well, and that makes us less likely to eat right, exercise, and enjoy sex the way we're supposed to—all the things that keep us feeling at the top of our game.

The good news is that Mother Nature is smarter than all the 21st-century health risks we face, and she has engineered many ways for us to fight this damage—just by picking up our forks. Even though antioxidant research is still a relatively new field, researchers have already identified hundreds of these healthy compounds in the foods we eat, and many researchers believe that there are likely thousands of these beneficial micronutrients.

I like to picture antioxidants as little molecules flying through our bloodstreams, wearing capes like superheroes (I do have a 6-year-old boy, after all!). The vast majority of these "free-radical fighters" are found in plants—including fruits, vegetables, and delicious whole grains—and in healthy fats like nuts. Small amounts, though, are in other healthy foods, which you'll also be getting plenty of on the O$_2$ Diet: fish, eggs, and dairy.

To me, the bummer is that the average person—looking to lower cholesterol, increase energy, and, of course, be thin—doesn't know much about any of these foods. Sure, people can talk about Splenda, Lipitor, or high-fructose corn syrup. But ask them what makes a walnut wonderful and they draw a blank. It's disconcerting that we've deprived ourselves of the natural protections found in food, often in the name of maintaining a healthy weight: Most people are stunned when I tell them

Your O$_2$ Moment:
Two things to try today

1. Settle down in a comfortable chair with a cup of green tea while reading this book. An 8-ounce mug has 3,000 ORAC points.

2. Take 10 deep breaths, counting your exhalations. Neuroscientists have confirmed that people who meditate have significantly lower levels of oxidative stress damage.[2] Yes—that means fewer free radicals.

that obese people are more likely to be deficient in key micronutrients, or that 25 percent of all menstruating women routinely deprive themselves of enough iron,[3] compromising the body's ability to fend off oxidative damage. And yes, that deprivation absolutely contributes to their risk for diseases, decreased energy level, and signs of aging—not to mention their constant struggle to control their appetite.

My plan isn't about popping pills or zero-this and zero-that foods. It's not about avoiding bad foods. It is about eating—eating *more* real food! By learning to crank up the number of foods that are high on the ORAC scale, you'll feel *better*. You'll have all the energy you need but be able to relax when you want. You'll feel strong and focused—you'll be in the zone! Will all those tempting lousy foods disappear from your radar forever? Sorry, no—I can't rid the world of curly fries and cupcakes. But the changes you'll notice in the way you look and feel will be so significant that unhealthy choices will be much less enticing.

Eating more of the right foods may seem like a subtle shift, but it's not: When you realize you have the power to boost your health with every food choice you make, you'll see that daily 4:00 p.m. struggle with the vending machine's salty chips in a whole new light. (You know the cycle I'm talking about. You either eat the chips, feel bad, then overeat at dinner because the whole day is ruined. Or you resist the chips, feel bad, and then overeat at dinner because you feel deprived.) Once you understand the variety and the power of ORAC foods, your idea of splurging will shift from utterly uninspired junk food to a handful of delicate, fresh blackberries or a tablespoon of tangy tomato sauce with fresh herbs.

My hope for you is that as you follow the O₂ Diet, you'll develop a brand-new philosophy of eating, one that is so much bigger than the struggle between you and that bag of potato chips. I know it sounds a little corny, but you will begin to realize that just as you are the author of your own life, you are also your own personal wellness coach. That means you are your body's best caretaker and guardian, not someone who wants to sabotage it with empty calories. I love to eat, too, and even I am not immune to the wrong kinds of foods—my personal weakness is chocolate-chip cookies, straight out of the oven. But for the most part,

I see food as an opportunity to nourish, and it's very satisfying for me to see people "flip the switch" on their own thinking.

The more success you have with the O₂ Diet—the more energy, compliments, and weight loss you reap, combined with the delightful realization that you actually *like* to work out and *like* healthy food—the more this diet will become second nature. Bonus: I can even promise you this plan will make your sex life better. How many diets can do that?

where ORAC numbers come from

Even the most sophisticated *nutritionistas*—the ones who spend hours at the local Whole Foods Market, for example, and who have 32 recipes for wheat berries—don't know much about the ORAC scale. ORAC is a method of measuring a food's potential to control those single oxygen molecules (free radicals).

The first ORAC test was developed in the early 1990s by Dr. Guohua Cao, a physician and chemist with the National Institute on Aging in Baltimore. Since then, Cao and dozens of other scientists, working at the US Department of Agriculture, such universities as the Jean Mayer USDA Human Nutrition Research Center on Aging at Tufts University in Boston (my alma mater!), and many commercial labs, have been refining the test. (The USDA's list, which ranks the ORAC values of 277 foods, is considered to be the most definitive; with a few exceptions, those are the ORAC scores I've built the O₂ Diet around.)

The ORAC scale offers a fairly precise measure of the ability of a given food, supplement, or compound to either destroy or neutralize the disease-causing free radicals. The test, which can be done on foods, tissue, or living plasma, actually takes two measurements into account—one of hydrophilic antioxidants (which just means chemicals that bond with water) and one of lipophilic antioxidants (those that bond best with fats)—to come up with a single score. That's the number I'll use for each food throughout the book.

So far, some of the foods that have proven to be the most powerful are on the obscure side (I admit it—even I didn't know what to do with maca

Why 30,000?

Researchers have just begun to scratch the surface of antioxidant research; there are now literally hundreds of studies linking antioxidant-rich foods to better health, including everything from reduced heart disease to a decreased likelihood of cancer. And while taking too many antioxidant supplements in pill form may be harmful, there's absolutely no downside to consuming more nutrient-dense fruits and vegetables. Although the current recommendations are that we eat between 3,000 and 5,000 ORAC points a day for optimum health, why not get all you can? As long as you are not overconsuming calories, you can have as many points as you want. The O$_2$ Diet is built around consuming 30,000 ORAC points a day.

Think that number sounds crazy? It's not unrealistic at all. If you eat the high-ORAC fruits, vegetables, and other foods I recommend, all within a range of calories that will allow you to achieve your healthiest weight, it's not tough to achieve the number.

Don't forget that you still need to eat a balanced diet. Sure, you could get to 30,000 easily on nothing but artichokes, blueberries, and hot cocoa. But that's not a balanced diet, and you'd be cheating yourself out of the wide variety of nutrients out there.

at first!). Others—like acai juice, goji berries, and pomegranate juice—are becoming more widely available. And finding the next "superfood" has become an obsession for many nutrition researchers. In fact, some companies have gotten a little carried away with these claims, and almost daily I need to warn clients away from some quack product they found on the Internet. Some of these new superfoods are super, but if they sound too good to be true, they probably are.

But the majority of the research—and I don't mean a few articles here and there, but hundreds of well-respected studies, conducted at leading universities—has shown that the most powerful foods are also among the most common. They're the foods your mother and grandmother always told you to eat. Of course, Mom (and our other ancestors) may not have known why green leafy vegetables, broccoli, squash, berries, and nuts were so important, but our forebears did a much better job of getting enough of those foods than we do. As much as I love learning about exotic new foods from faraway places, introducing them to my family, and recommending them to clients, I still get jazzed about the research that substantiates the healthy food choices people have been making for centuries, and about the fact that plain old apples are one of the best antioxidant foods around: A single Granny Smith packs almost 7,100 ORAC points. Thank you, Benjamin Franklin!

the next frontier

Is the ORAC scale perfect? No scientific measure is perfect. It's important to keep in mind that, relatively speaking, antioxidant research is still in its infancy. Although researchers were working to understand the oxidative process of metals as early as the 19th century, the focus on antioxidants in nutrition is thought to have gotten under way in 1926, when a team of scientists identified carotene—the orangish, vitamin A–rich chemical that gives cantaloupe, apricots, and sweet potatoes their antioxidant power. Antioxidant research took off in the 1980s as researchers focused on antioxidants in vitamin supplements, and in the 1990s, researchers turned to studying antioxidants that naturally occur in foods.

What variables affect a food's ORAC value? Let's take blueberries as an example. Just because a cup of blueberries earns a score of 9,700 points in the USDA's lab, that's no guarantee that the cup of blueberries you have in your kitchen right now will have the same value. The berries were grown in different soil, from different cultivars, using different fertilizers, and were even harvested at different times of year—any of those

Your O_2 Injection:
Start right now!

Even if you're not yet ready to start the kickoff phase of the O_2 Diet, you can start feeling healthier right away. Beginning tomorrow morning (or today!), drink a large glass of water with 1 ounce of lemon juice, eliminate all added salt and sugar, and eat 1 cup of blueberries and 1 cup of cooked kale at some point during the day..

factors may cause variations. Or think about the broccoli in your fridge. It probably degraded for a week or so traveling in the truck from California and then sitting in your store's produce aisle, and it may not score as highly as frozen broccoli flash frozen within hours of being picked. (For that matter, I can't promise you that the hard-boiled egg you just ate has 76 calories, only that, on average, most eggs do.)

Nor can any researcher promise you that the antioxidant foods I recommend are the most potent. Perhaps one day we could learn that the lycopene in a tomato is responsible for even more health benefits than we know about today. And it's just as possible that one morning we'll pick up *USA Today* and read about a brand-new antioxidant, a superstar compound that trumps every other phytonutrient we know of. To me, that is what makes nutrition so exciting—researchers crank out a steady stream of new evidence and information that makes our food choices more informed than ever.

James Joseph, PhD, a leading researcher at the Jean Mayer USDA Human Nutrition Research Center on Aging at Tufts University, tells me he believes that the next few years we will see big breakthroughs in our understanding of the precise ways that fruits work, including finding the brain receptors for compounds like polyphenols, as well as the ways the antioxidants from certain foods may replace commonly prescribed drugs. "As long as you consume antioxidants in food, you can't overdo it," he explains. "It's very important to get a variety of antioxidants." His personal favorites are blueberries, walnuts, and a little dark chocolate every day.

Sounds good, doesn't it? The delicious foods and rapidly evolving science behind the O_2 Diet reinforce the reasons for respecting the potency of healthy foods and choosing foods wisely as often as possible, every single day. The funny part? For all those people looking for a quick fix or a magic pill to solve their problems—from wrinkles to sagging boobs to a weight problem or a flat tush or high blood pressure—this is it! In just 32 days, this back-to-basics approach to eating will make you feel and look better than any vitamin pill, Botox injection, or 12 more sessions with that personal trainer.

2

Health Benefits You Can See Now, Foods You Can Love Forever

I bet you are a weight-loss warrior. You know what I mean: You've spent years with your fists up, ready to battle that scale every morning, poring over the latest celebrity weight-loss saga, or counting to 10 in the hope that the craving will pass and you'll find the strength to just say no to bad foods. So what I'm asking you to do is not easy! Instead of seeing the world as a place where sneaky foods are trying to sabotage you and force you into pants with elastic waistbands, I'm encouraging you to look at life as a place with an abundance of healthy options. Supermarkets, restaurants, airports, and, yes, even vending machines usually offer something that is truly good for you. Every bite, every meal, every snack you consume is an opportunity for you to become healthier. In short, I want you to start thinking of your fork as your body's new best friend—not as the enemy waiting to stab you.

As weird as it may sound, I want you to stop thinking about what you're trying to *prevent*, whether it's weight gain or high cholesterol. Instead, I need you to picture exactly what you are trying to *build*. I tell my clients every day to "flip the switch": Focus on what you *can* do for your body, not what you can't do or have. Once you flip that switch, you'll get excited about eating in a new way. You will think about foods and beverages as choices that, yes, can help you lose weight. But you'll also see them as the raw materials for creating a healthier body and glowing skin, for providing you with the energy and focus you need to get through your busy day.

The O_2 Diet is based on foods that will help you achieve your ideal weight *and* help you function better than you ever have. This diet does much more than provide the basic calories you need to make it until bedtime. It offers more genuine *nutrition* than you probably have eaten in your entire life. Consuming the O_2 Diet's 30,000 ORAC points each day will certainly help you reach your target weight. But this diet also steers you toward the best foods for addressing your other health concerns. Some foods have been shown to be beneficial in easing the outward signs of aging, for example, while others are proven boosters for the immune system.

I am giving you the power—and the tools—to be your own dietitian. If your family tree is plagued with heart disease, I hope you'll pay special attention to the foods I list in this chapter's "Foods for a Healthier Heart" section. If one of your main complaints is that you feel constantly scatterbrained or anxious, you may benefit from the antioxidant foods researchers have found to be especially beneficial to cognitive functioning—see "Foods for a Focused Mind." Skin looking dull and blotchy? There are specific foods for addressing that, too!

I've recommended my favorite foods in each health category based not just on the latest antioxidant research but also on my clinical experience with what people like to eat best. Don't be surprised when some of these potent foods crop up over and over, because they have many active ingredients and serve many functions. Grapes, for example, have at least 15 known antioxidant compounds, ranging from the much-discussed resveratrol to quercetin to pectin to vitamin C! So while I can confidently recommend grapes to boost your heart health, I also get psyched about the fact that grapes will likely be good for your brain and your skin, too. It also means you can indulge in that glass of red wine by the fire—I am all about efficiency!

In short, all of those foods are what I consider healthy *plus,* and it's a good idea for everyone to eat *more* of them. Don't worry about tallying up ORAC points right now—you'll meet these foods and see their associated ORAC points frequently in this book, worked into my delicious recipes, given as options in my do-it-yourself plan, and featured on my shopping list. In the glossary, I also give a brief description of the chemical components scientists believe make these foods so special. Also, note that some of the foods listed below have ORAC points associated with them and some do not. This is because not all foods have been tested. This doesn't mean that they do not contain any ORAC value, nor does it mean that there aren't many other healthy nutrients in the food as well!

foods for a slimmer body

These are some of the weight-loss wonders that make the O₂ Diet so effective. (You'll get the nitty-gritty details on losing weight with the diet in the next chapter.)

Almonds Crunch your way back into your favorite jeans! For years, experts have said that a calorie is a calorie is a calorie. But when researchers kept two groups of dieters on the same number of calories daily, giving one group almonds each day, the almond eaters lost more weight than the other group.[1] We can credit the almonds' healthy fat and vitamin E. I think these nuts are a dieter's best friend because they taste great and leave us with a sense of *satiety*—one of my favorite words and the technical term for feeling full and happy. A 10-almond serving provides about 600 ORAC points.

Artichokes What's more fun to eat than steamed artichokes? I love them because they're one of the best calorie bargains going, at 60 calories each. Eat an artichoke as an appetizer and you may end up consuming fewer calories overall at the meal. Artichokes are also superhigh on the ORAC scale—7,900 ORAC points—and they contain phytochemicals that may lower cholesterol levels and act as an anti-inflammatory in the skin, making them a beauty food as well.

Your weight-loss goal, plus . . .

How much weight you lose in the next 32 days depends on your goals and your current habits. If you're already an oatmeal-loving gym junkie, it will take you longer to lose weight than if you've got six weekly visits to Burger King you can cut out.

Write down your goal, then weigh yourself weekly:

Starting weight _____ Date _____

32-day weight-loss goal _____

After 4-day cleanse _____ Date _____

After week 1 _____ Date _____

After week 2 _____ Date _____

After week 3 _____ Date _____

After week 4 _____ Date _____

But don't stop there—choose one other goal. Better skin? Less stress? A healthier heart?

Write it down: _____
Then make a conscious effort to eat foods that will support that goal every single day for the next month.

Chile peppers These bright red peppers, which fuel the fire in cayenne pepper, contain an antioxidant called capsaicin. While the substance gets a lot of attention for its medical applications and is even used as a topical pain reliever, it also seems to have some effect on human appetite. Some studies have found that people who eat meals with plenty of this delicious (and hot!) spice feel less hungry as a result.

Fatty fish On the one hand, you'll hear me talk a lot about *lean* protein sources as being vital to your weight-loss success. But I also tout *fatty* fish—like salmon, mackerel, and sardines—because of their plentiful calcium, vitamin D stores, and omega-3 fatty acids, which you'll hear more about later. Besides their many health benefits, fatty fish have been shown to prevent weight gain in women.

Flaxseed The best reason ever to head to your local health food store, these powerful little seeds have a nice, nutty flavor. While the whole seed is harder to digest, in its ground-up form, flax provides a dynamite dietary source of lignans, plant estrogens that may soothe the monthly mood swings that can lead to emotional overeating. My favorite flaxseed mix, which is on the shopping list (page 176), even contains blueberries, strawberries, and cranberries.

Green tea Move over, java—even coffee lovers need to learn to make time for this fat-melting tea. While white, black, oolong, and green teas all come from the same plant and have similar amounts of caffeine, green tea leaves are prepared differently. Green tea leaves aren't fermented before drying, and they provide about 3,000 ORAC points per cup. As a result, green tea is richer in antioxidants called catechins, which may trigger weight loss by stimulating the body to burn calories and decrease body fat. Buy tea bags in small quantities, though, and store in their original packaging, out of the sun: Studies have found that green tea bags can lose up to 32 percent of their antioxidant power in 6 months.[2]

Lemon water Pucker up, my friends: Starting off your day with a glass of lemon water, and drinking enough of it throughout the day, helps with weight loss in several ways. First, there's an emotional component—it's a simple, subtle step that makes you feel empowered and that will spur you to make good choices for the rest of the day. Second, researchers have long known that dieters who replace sweetened drinks with water lose weight more quickly than those who don't. Many people overeat because they are actually thirsty and just can't tell the difference between thirst and hunger. Loading up on water, especially earlier in the day, prevents that. When you're adequately hydrated, your metabolism functions at its best. And lemon peels— besides offering a fresh and tangy flavor—contain pectin, which has been shown to help with weight loss. Add an ounce of lemon juice (and some zest, too!) to each of your 8 daily glasses of water and you'll add 3,200 ORAC points.

Lentils For people looking to lose weight, lentils are real superheroes. Like all other legumes, they provide lean protein, which gives your metabolism a little boost as soon as you eat, helping you burn more calories throughout the day. They contain plenty of fiber, which keeps you feeling full, and they have impressive amounts of B vitamins, iron, and zinc. But what makes them so much better than other beans is that they can be prepared quickly—you can have a delicious meal ready in less than 45 minutes, compared to hours for other legumes. My favorite? Black lentils, which are sometimes called beluga because they glisten and shine like caviar once they're cooked. A ½-cup serving has 7,500 ORAC points.

Red grapefruit This is more than a breakfast food—it's a weight-loss jump start! Packed with vitamin C and fiber, this citrus fruit speeds weight loss. One study found that people who ate half a grapefruit with each meal lost 3.6 pounds, while those who drank a serving of grapefruit juice three times a day lost 3.3 pounds.[3] (Many people in the study lost more than 10 pounds—without making any other dietary changes.) Even if these claims are too good to be true, I have a soft spot for grapefruit—I grew up eating a half grapefruit before dinner every single night. While all grapefruit is great, the pink and red varieties contain lycopene and are extragood for your heart. Half a grapefruit has 1,900 ORAC points.

Turnips No, they're not glamorous. But they're great vegetables for dieters to have on hand—not only do turnips keep well, but they're always available in supermarkets and are an excellent source of complex carbs, which keep you satisfied longer because they have both soluble and insoluble fiber. Turnips also contain an unexpectedly high amount of vitamin C. If you live in a cooler climate, you can also experiment with rutabagas, a close relative of the turnip.

Yogurt One of my go-to snacks, yogurt has healthy bacteria that keep digestion efficient, a must for anyone trying to shed pounds. Research has shown that people who consume plenty of low-fat dairy products are able to lose more weight than people who don't.[4]

foods for an amazing appearance

One of the reasons researchers have vigorously pursued most antioxidants is to prevent disease. But honestly, the quest for ageless beauty plays a big role, too—what scientist wouldn't like to be the one to discover the fountain of youth, the magic bullet that could make us all look like we were 20 again? I'll admit it: The first time I noticed some lines around my mouth—as much as I like to think it's because I smile so much—I panicked a little!

There aren't any foods that will turn back the clock—at least, not that we know of yet. (Believe me, if we ever find such a food, I'll be first in line.) But there *are* foods that can make you look much better and slow down the aging process:

Cantaloupe This fruit helps anyone with a sweet tooth fend off cravings, and it's also a nutrient bonanza. A single serving of this delicious melon provides you with more than your Recommended Dietary Allowance (RDA) of vitamin A. And of course, most of us are aware that vitamin A products are good for the skin when applied topically—it's what gives products like Retin-A their stop-the-clock power. But *consuming* enough dietary vitamin A is essential for preventing a dry, flaky complexion. Melons also have plenty of vitamins B_3, B_6, and C. Besides promoting healthy cell turnover and aiding in the formation of collagen and elastin, vitamin C is key in countering the effects of sun damage.

You can cut the melon into pieces and refrigerate; the refrigerated fruit won't lose its nutritional benefits. One cup has 500 ORAC points.

Coconut This tropical wonder does more than make a good piña colada: Coconut improves the absorption of the minerals calcium and magnesium. Since these nutrients are crucial for a gorgeous grin, coconut is vital. And it doesn't hurt that coconut's medium-chain triglycerides help burn fat! Try swapping out peanut butter for 2 teaspoons of coconut butter on a high-fiber cracker for a delicious snack.

Figs I'm in awe of figs from a purely nutritional standpoint. A recent study, for example, found that a handful of dried figs increased people's antioxidant plasma level for 4 hours (much longer than many foods), and that was enough to offset the oxidative damage done by a carbonated soft drink![5] Since biblical times, figs have been considered a topical beauty treatment; they contain alpha hydroxy acids that help exfoliate skin (more about that later). But the real reason I think of them as a beauty food is their heavenly smell—can you say "Garden of Eden"?—that makes everyone feel relaxed and serene. Two small figs have about 2,700 ORAC points.

Honey Nature's antibacterial agent! Used on your skin, this beauty food is good for treating acne and reducing redness. It's also a natural humectant, which means it keeps all that water you're drinking in the right places. When you eat honey, its antibacterial, antiviral, and antifungal properties protect you, too. And daily consumption boosts the level of polyphenolic antioxidants in the blood.

Lean proteins, including beef, chicken, and fish No, they don't star in any topical spa treatment—at least, that's one chicken wrap I never want to see! But these foods contain coenzyme Q10, also called ubiquinone, which has antioxidant properties that are powerful in fighting aging and that help skin cells renew properly. This antioxidant, which your body can also manufacture on its own, is appearing in more and more skin products, too, because it's a small molecule that's easily absorbed.

Lobster While most people think of lobster as a major splurge, prices fluctuate, making these delicious critters downright affordable from time to time. And besides keeping you slim—they're an impressive source of protein, with only a gram of fat per serving—they're also beauty bonanzas, providing plenty of vitamin B_{12} and zinc, which help keep our skin looking great. Live in the South? Crawfish are just as good for you.

Mushrooms While brightly colored vegetables get much of the attention in antioxidant news, these fungi are emerging as nutritional steamrollers, providing B_6, folate, niacin, riboflavin, iron, potassium, and selenium. Once you start dabbling in 'shrooms, you'll be amazed at the variety—there are more than 35,000 kinds, although many of them are extremely poisonous. Most of us grew up eating button mushrooms, but branch out and try deliciously woodsy maitake, or hen-of-the-woods; melt-in-your-mouth oyster mushrooms; or the more strongly flavored shiitake. And yep, they're a true beauty food: In ancient times, Chinese women ate them for a smooth complexion, and you'll find mushroom extracts in many high-end beauty products.

Olive oil It tastes great, and it's so good for you. Besides being among the healthiest types of fats, olive oil tends to be rich in polyphenols, which aren't just antioxidants—they're also antifungal and antibacterial agents. Eating olive oil is great, but you can put it right on your skin, too. I like to mix it with a little avocado, apply, and leave it on for 10 minutes. It's so nourishing, you can almost feel your skin drinking it up! A 2-teaspoon serving, when eaten, has about 100 ORAC points.

Oysters These low-cal, high-protein sea creatures contain zinc, which has antioxidant properties, keeps your hair shining, and is especially important if you're prone to acne. (Since oysters are also said to be an aphrodisiac, eating them with your sweetheart might be enough to make you start looking sexier!)

Papayas Another tropical treat, these bright orange fruits contain vitamins A, C, and E and papain, a digestive enzyme that is a mild exfoliant. When you eat papayas, these chemical compounds don't only help your skin look better—they're also good for your eyes, heart, and immune system. We've already explained how essential vitamin C is for skin, but vitamin E is also vital, and an important way the body wards off sun damage, such as age spots and wrinkles. One cup has 500 ORAC points.

Your O₂ Breakthrough:
What all antioxidants have in common

There are so many different kinds of antioxidants—at least 4,000 flavonoids alone—that it's easy to get the idea that experts toss the word around carelessly. How could a chemical like an anthocyanin, found in abundance in blueberries, be considered the same thing as, let's say, alpha-lipoic acid, an antioxidant chemical the body creates all on its own? How can it be that just a few vitamins and minerals act as antioxidants, but not all of them do?

Great questions! The answer is that these wide varieties of compounds don't have much in common in terms of their chemical makeup. What puts them all under the enormous antioxidant umbrella is what they *do*, not what they are. While each compound may accomplish the job in different ways, any substance called an antioxidant has been shown to minimize the effect of those highly reactive free radicals created by stress, pollution, aging, and illness.

Quinoa Granted, quinoa is not exactly a household name yet—but it should be. An excellent source of the vitamin B complex, this nutty grain keeps skin cells repairing themselves. If you don't get your Bs, you will have scaly, dry skin, and sometimes even hair loss.

Red bell peppers I love the way these juicy, crunchy vegetables taste. I can snack on strips of them endlessly. Fresh red bell peppers have a higher antioxidant capacity than other types of peppers and higher amounts of vitamin C (providing more than 450 percent of the RDA), vitamin A, vitamin B_6, vitamin E, fiber, and other antioxidants. The unique combination of large amounts of vitamins A, C, and E makes red bell peppers a superfood for your skin. A half cup—the amount you'd toss into a normal salad—adds 600 ORAC points.

Rosemary Who doesn't love the way this pungent herb smells? But that isn't the only reason it appears in so many hair and body products: Whether we eat it or use it topically, the fragrant oils stimulate circulation and act as an anti-irritant. One teaspoon has 400 ORAC points.

Salmon Besides its weight-loss benefit, salmon reduces inflammation, calming the skin and making it glow.

Strawberries Smile! These berries contain malic acid, which acts as an astringent to remove surface discoloration from your teeth. A 1-cup serving provides 5,400 ORAC points.

Watermelon This lycopene-rich fruit provides 33 percent more protection against sunburn than other fruits. (Sorry, you still have to wear sunscreen—but isn't it nice to know your snack is protecting your skin, too?) One cup of diced melon has 300 ORAC points.

foods for a healthier body— fight cancer, boost immune function, and strengthen bones

Certain antioxidants have been shown to fight cancer, others to boost immunity, and still others to help keep muscles and bones strong. My faves:

Avocados I seriously *feel* healthier when I am in the kitchen slicing an avocado. Rich in glutathione, a substance that specifically blocks intestinal absorption of certain fats that cause oxidative damage, these fruits also contain lutein, beta-carotene, and vitamin E. And by all means, bring on the salsa—Ohio State University researchers say that combining avocado with other foods may allow for better absorption of the antioxidants in those foods.[6] A single serving (about one-quarter of an avocado) contains about 700 ORAC points.

Beans Because so many of my clients want to lose weight, beans are a favorite part of my arsenal—they're high in fiber and full of lean protein, and they leave you feeling satisfied for hours. They are also loaded with phytochemicals (including saponins, protease inhibitors, and phytic acid), which appear to protect our cells from damage that can lead to cancer, reports the American Institute for Cancer Research (AICR). A half-cup serving of black beans, one of the tastiest varieties, contains 8,000 ORAC points. Make all the jokes you want about beans giving you gas—as long as you gradually work your way up to consuming larger amounts of any high-fiber food, you won't kill the romance!

Broccoli, cabbage, and cauliflower Don't laugh, but I think of broccoli as the Brad Pitt of vegetables—it improves just about any meal! These cruciferous vegetables (which also include brussels sprouts, bok choy, and kale) are low-calorie cancer fighters, says the AICR. Researchers at the University of California at Berkeley have found that some of the compounds in broccoli boost the immune system, doubling the number of white blood cells. Sulforaphane, another chemical found in broccoli, helps us breathe easier, minimizing free-radical damage in the lungs. A serving of broccoli contains 600 ORAC points.

Cilantro This herb is one of those love-it-or-hate-it foods, which is why so many Mexican restaurants serve both "with" and "without" versions of guacamole. Technically a dark, leafy vegetable, it has beta-carotene and plenty of vitamins, including A and K. It also contains a natural antibiotic, which may help in warding off illness.

Coffee I have been known to bring coffee with me on the elliptical trainer, and that first cup of coffee is right up there with my kids' a.m. kisses as my favorite part of the day. Coffee gets a bad rap, mostly because people abuse it (drinking more than the suggested 2 to 3 cups daily is linked to certain health problems) or because they load it up with sugary and artificial additives. But it's a leading source of antioxidants for most Americans, and researchers have found that coffee drinkers have a lower risk of developing type 2 diabetes, perhaps because of the antioxidant known as chlorogenic acid. Coffee is also what experts call an ergogenic, meaning it enhances physical performance. Don't believe me? Try a cup of coffee about an hour before your next workout and see if you don't feel a difference. (Want to know more about coffee? See the box on page 30.)

Eggs Talk about the perfect package! Eggs are affordable, low in calories, and a versatile protein (not to mention a big source of choline, which we need for healthy brain function). They also contain lutein and zeaxanthin, antioxidants that researchers say are linked to healthy eyesight.

Garlic and onions Go ahead, have bad breath! Garlic, onions, scallions, leeks, and chives are all part of the *Allium* genus and likely protect us against stomach cancer; garlic has been especially linked with lower rates of colorectal cancer. In lab studies,[7] the antioxidant components (including allicin, allixin, allyl sulfides, quercetin, and a large group of organosulfur compounds) have shown the ability to slow or stop the growth of tumors in prostate, bladder, colon, and stomach tissue. One serving has about 150 ORAC points. One cup of onions has 1,600 ORAC points.

Ginger I love it for its zingy flavor, but ginger is also an impressive anti-inflammatory and deserves a front-and-center spot on your spice rack. And there's a reason your mom let you sip ginger ale when you felt sick—this spice is a winner for treating car sickness, nausea, and even morning sickness. One teaspoon of ginger has 500 ORAC points.

Okra When cooked the wrong way, okra makes a memorable impression—*slimy* is the only word that describes it! But when cooked right—don't wash the okra until just before you plan to cook it!—it's delicious, and the ooze that comes from the sliced vegetable is what thickens delicious sauces and stews. Come on, who can resist a good gumbo? While okra is hard to find fresh all year round, frozen okra tastes just as good, and because it's particularly rich in soluble fiber, experts believe it can help lower your LDL cholesterol level. But I think of it as an all-around health booster, because it provides a wealth of B vitamins, vitamin C, magnesium, and potassium, as well as lutein and zeaxanthin, both important members of the beta-carotene family.

Persimmons In some parts of Asia, this fruit is even more popular than oranges! And with its flashy orange-red skin, it always catches my eye when it starts arriving in the produce aisle in the fall. That color, in fact, is why we should all eat more persimmons—these juicy fruits are packed with alpha-carotene, beta-carotene, and beta-cryptoxanthin, not to mention plenty of vitamin C, a key immune booster.

Pineapple Just a whiff of this fruit is enough to give me a flashback to a tropical island. But pineapple is a nutrition standout: It's the only known source of bromelain, an enzyme whose anti-inflammatory properties may ease joint pain. Research also suggests it helps heal injuries, reduce the inflammation associated with asthma, and slow the growth of some cancers. The sweet variety of pineapple averages about 1,500 ORAC points per serving.

Prunes Okay, so they're not pretty. But these wrinkly little fruits are rich in vitamin K and a top source of the mineral boron, and we need both for strong bones. Researchers have found that prunes provide protection against postmenopausal bone loss.[8] One three-prune serving gives you 1,900 ORAC points.

Soy You don't have to be a vegan to love soy! Everyone should swap a meal of meat for a vegetarian dish a few times a week: It's good for your health and for the planet. I'm a big fan of soy foods not just because they are tasty but because they are so easy to work into your meal plan. Whether it's soy milk or tasty edamame, somewhere there's a version of soy with your name on it. While soy is not without controversy, it's emerging as a powerful component of a healthy diet, with the AICR reporting that its active ingredients—such as isoflavones (which have been studied most), saponins, phenolic acids, phytic acid, and phytosterols—have anticancer properties. A half-cup serving of soybeans adds 5,400 ORAC points to your salad.

Spinach and kale Talk about all-stars: These two leafy greens—as well as others like romaine lettuce, red leaf lettuce, mustard greens, collard greens, chicory, and Swiss chard—are excellent sources of fiber, folate, and a wide range of carotenoids, likely providing protection against cancers of the mouth, pharynx, larynx, and pancreas and slowing the growth of some types of breast, skin, lung, and stomach cancer cells. Experts believe that carotenoids seem to prevent cancer by acting as antioxidants—that is, by scouring potentially dangerous free radicals from the body before they can do harm. Another bonus is that carotenoids have been proven to slow sarcopenia—that's the fancy name for the natural damage that occurs to our muscles as we age. One cup of easy-to-prepare frozen spinach provides about 2,600 ORAC points.

Sweet potato Like most people, I've got a little bit of a sweet tooth. A medium baked sweet potato not only satisfies that craving but also contains over 400 percent of the RDA of vitamin A and more eye-healthy beta-carotene than any other fruit or vegetable. A baked sweet potato, with its skin, provides 2,400 ORAC points.

foods for a healthier heart

Younger women tend to be oblivious to the risks of heart disease—I know, you're thinking that heart disease happens only to, ahem, *older* people. But that attitude itself is a big risk. Heart disease continues to be the number-one killer in the United States—even among women. How you eat *today* will predict how healthy your heart is 30 years from now. And yes, heart health is directly related to oxidative damage: The oxidation of low-density lipoprotein (LDL, or "bad" cholesterol) is what causes fatty buildups in the arteries—a condition called atherosclerosis, which can lead to heart attacks and strokes.

Some experts believe that taking antioxidants in a supplement form may help stop this gunk from forming in our pipes. You may have also seen studies that have found that these pills may not protect the heart and may even create some health risks. Remember, nutrition is a new science and we will constantly hear of new research—that is what makes it so exciting. The American Heart Association recommends a diet high in food sources of antioxidants and other heart-protecting nutrients, such as fruits, vegetables, whole grains, and nuts—I am a nutritionist, so of course I agree we need to get nutrients from food! We should get our nutrients from food and that is what this book is all about but I also agree with the AHA and other medical experts, including the American Medical Association, that taking a multivitamin each day is good insurance against deficiencies; after all, we all have days when we just don't eat well at all! I recommend my clients take a multivitamin for insurance as well as other supplements depending on their needs—again, as back up support to a healthy diet. Check with a registered dietitian or your doctor to see what is right for you. You can also go to www.theO2diet. com for more complete list of supplements I recommend.

Asparagus All greens are great. Even though it may turn your urine bright yellow and make it smell funny, asparagus has the special honor of being extrahigh in folate, which is essential for a healthy cardiovascular system. Half a cup adds 2,900 ORAC points to your daily level and is a big boost for heart health. No wonder ancient Egyptians considered it food for the gods!

Capers Not only are these delicious little nuggets—technically, unopened flower buds of the caper plant—rich in an antioxidant called rutin, but researchers believe that when as few as a tablespoonful are served with meat, they counteract harmful digestive by-products that have been linked to cancer risks. Researchers think capers contain a substance that prevents the oxidative damage meats can cause.

Cherries University of Michigan researchers have found that the anthocyanins in dark cherries, especially the tarter varieties, reduce inflammation and lower cholesterol and triglyceride levels; they pack 3,500 ORAC points per serving.[9] Just don't swallow the pits!

Dark chocolate See, you always knew there was a reason chocolate could make you swoon! Rich in flavonoids, chocolate is believed to promote heart health by reducing platelet activation, affecting the relaxation capabilities of blood vessels, and it may also affect the balance of certain hormonelike compounds called eicosanoids, which are thought to play a role in cardiovascular health, reports the Cleveland Clinic. Don't be shocked that I think dark chocolate can be part of a weight-loss plan: The fat in chocolate isn't as bad as most people think. One ounce of dark chocolate has 5,900 ORAC points, and some companies (such as Xoçai) are making chocolate with more than that. A single serving (three nuggets) of Xoçai has 10,700 ORAC points and just 100 calories.

Fish It's not just for slimming down. The American Heart Association recommends eating fish such as salmon, trout, or herring at least twice a week; recent research shows that eating these oily swimmers, which contain omega-3 fatty acids, may help lower your risk of death from coronary artery disease.[10]

Grapes The darker the skin, the better. Those phenol compounds—including resveratrol and quercetin—reduce inflammation and promote a healthy heart. Most red grapes have 1,200 ORAC points per serving.

Hibiscus tea Another great reason to celebrate afternoon teatime! A Tufts University study found that people with borderline high blood pressure who drank 3 cups a day of hibiscus-rich herbal teas (I like Celestial Seasonings Red Zinger) lowered their blood pressure by 7 points—sometimes almost back to normal.[11]

Oregano To an extent, all herbs and spices are heart healthy: The more we use them, the less likely we are to reach for the saltshaker, and lowering sodium intake is key to keeping blood pressure in check. But oregano is by far the most antioxidant-dense spice, ranking highest of all 27 tested by the USDA. On a per-gram basis, it has four times more antioxidant activity than blueberries do! One of the antioxidants oregano contains is beta-caryophyllene, a substance that reduces inflammation, which can lead to heart disease. And while most of us learned to prize it on our pizza, it's a nice touch for just about any Italian- or Mexican-inspired recipe. One teaspoon of dried oregano has 3,600 ORAC points.

Pecans I stow nuts everywhere—in my desk drawers, my backpack, and even my evening bags. All nuts tend to be rich in vitamin E, a powerful antioxidant, as well as a good source of protein and heart-healthy fats. (Plus they're so satisfying that working them into your diet as, let's say, a mid-morning or mid-afternoon snack ensures you won't show up at your next meal hungry enough to eat the tablecloth.) Pecans have the highest antioxidant power and have been shown to reduce lipid oxidation—a critical measure of heart health—by 7.4 percent.[12] They also contain plant sterols, which lower cholesterol. Even the FDA agrees and suggests that eating 1.5 ounces of nuts, such as pecans, each day lowers the risk of heart disease. Eight halves contain 2,500 ORAC points.

Pistachios I have memories of my dad eating the red dyed ones while watching football. For many people, they're a great diet tool, since the time it takes to pop the little green guys out of their shells makes you eat them more slowly. And in many ways, they are nutritionally like other nuts, especially almonds. But pistachios are also packed with plant sterols, which researchers think lower the risk of heart disease. Eighteen pistachios has 1,000 ORAC points.

Quinces These pearlike fruits may not be popular in the United States, but they should be. Besides having lots of fiber and vitamin C, they also contain good amounts of pectin, which boosts heart health by lowering cholesterol. Quinces are usually available only in the winter months. Look for firm, fragrant, smooth fruit. While I've heard of people eating them raw, quinces are almost always served cooked. (I like them baked, like apples.)

Red wine Drink up, kid! While much of the research on wine has focused on the resveratrol in grapes, it seems something in the alcohol also raises high-density lipoprotein, or HDL, the "good" cholesterol. Major heart-health groups like the American Heart Association and the National Heart, Lung, and Blood Institute say that it's not a good idea to *start* drinking wine just to prevent heart disease: Alcohol can be addictive, is associated with other diseases, and has a fairly high calorie count. But if you do like to have a drink now and again, why not make it a 5-ounce serving of robust red wine? A nice Cabernet provides 7,400 ORAC points.

Tomatoes Besides having plenty of vitamin C, tomatoes are rich in lycopene. Researchers have found that the higher the serum level of this antioxidant found in people's blood, the lower the level of heart disease as well as other chronic illnesses.[13] A serving of three diced plum tomatoes adds 900 ORAC points to your day.

Winter squash While summer squash varieties, such as zucchini, are mostly water, hearty winter squash are teeming with complex carbs, beta-carotene, and lutein. But the high levels of both soluble and insoluble fiber mean they are cholesterol fighters, too. And best of all, they are one of the few low-fat sources of vitamin E.

foods for a focused mind

Much of what we know about the ways certain foods can help sharpen our minds comes from the field of Alzheimer's disease research. Once scientists made the connections between diet and dementia, they began to tease out the dietary components that protect against other neurological problems, providing us with plenty of insights on how eating better early in life can keep our thinking clearer as we age. I pay close attention to this research because Alzheimer's runs in my family, and the disease is heartbreaking. Anything we can do nutritionally to prevent or delay its onset fascinates me.

But all of us can sharpen neural functioning by eating more of the right kinds of foods. It turns out our brains and neural pathways are growing and improving all the time—not just when we're young. Yes, infants are growing at a much faster pace, sprouting billions of new nerve cells in the early years. But lower levels of growth continue throughout our lives. If we eat the right foods—including those antioxidants that seem to help our neural connections function at their best, such as coenzyme Q10, alpha-lipoic acid, ginkgo biloba, DHA (an omega-3 fatty acid), and vitamins C and E—we'll be able to concentrate better, remember more, and feel calmer.

My top choices to keep the brain focused, stress in check, and emotions balanced (God knows I need that daily!):

Black tea A cup of tea really *does* relieve stress: British researchers had two groups of people drink black tea four times a day for 6 weeks. Half of the group had real tea, and half had tea with all the active ingredients removed. The participants were then asked to perform stressful tasks. Fifty minutes after the task was over, the cortisol (a stress hormone) levels of real tea drinkers had dropped 47 percent, compared to just 27 percent for the fake tea. A cup contains about 2,700 ORAC points.

Blueberries All berries rock. But James Joseph, a leading antioxidant researcher, told me he thinks of these little powerhouses as the Hertz of fruits—number one with a bullet! Their antioxidant power comes from anthocyanins, which may lower LDL (lousy) cholesterol. Pectin, one of the soluble fibers in blueberries, also has cholesterol-lowering properties.

(Pectin helps keep you regular.) Blueberries show the most power when it comes to boosting memory, cognition, and balance. Researchers believe they do so by reducing inflammation and helping us overcome the normal effects of aging—all while providing 9,700 ORAC points per 1-cup serving.

Brazil nuts By now, you've figured out how much I like all nuts. But this variety has extrahigh levels of selenium. Without enough of this mineral, many people feel depressed, anxious, or irritable. Two brazil nuts will give you 100 ORAC points.

Cinnamon There's a reason most of us drool when we walk by a bakery, and cinnamon is a big part of it. Just the smell of this heavenly spice is enough to curb fatigue, ease frustration, and increase alertness.

Your O$_2$ Breakthrough:
The great java debate

Coffee—my morning beverage of choice, I'll admit!—is one of those things that health researchers have been squabbling about for decades.

Not that long ago, many experts encouraged people to cut down on coffee, or even eliminate it from their diets entirely. Experts thought it might be linked to heart disease, for example, and even some cancers, not to mention anxiety, insomnia, and general jitteriness. It contains high levels of caffeine, which is the most commonly used mood-altering drug in the world; on average, Americans drink 280 milligrams—the amount found in about 17 ounces of brewed coffee—each day. And once we're dependent, we're really dependent: Most people know that abruptly swearing off coffee can mean headaches and general fatigue.

But the latest research has swung in the opposite direction, and medical experts now believe that coffee helps *prevent* heart disease, stroke, and diabetes.

My advice? Listen to your body. If you are a coffee drinker and a couple of cups of coffee a day makes your life more pleasant, why give it up? Enjoy those extra antioxidants! But if you've noticed that you have trouble sleeping, or you've come to think of yourself as an anxious person, it may be time to experiment with cutting back a bit.

Also, make sure to enjoy those extra antioxidants without too many extra calories! Some of those frothy coffee creations Americans are guzzling by the tankerful? They can contain more than 1,000 calories apiece! So enjoy your coffee—but be very mindful of what you put in it. While black coffee has only a few calories, a

(Researchers tested it on stressed-out commuters as they drove.)[14] I cook with cinnamon as often as I can. Sometimes, on days when both my kids are screaming, I boil a cinnamon stick on the stove in the hope that its wonderful stress-busting aroma will keep me out of trouble! Besides managing stress, researchers believe cinnamon may inhibit certain types of Alzheimer's cells. When eaten, 1 teaspoon of cinnamon adds 7,000 ORAC points to a recipe.

Cottage cheese I love this creamy treat because it helps people get enough calcium, and the low-fat varieties are great protein sources, too. But it also rates high among good-mood foods because it has an unusually high level of the amino acid tryptophan, the same substance that makes turkey so soothing.

tablespoon of cream adds 50 calories, and a spoonful of sugar another 50. At your local java joint, a latte made with skim milk probably has 130 calories, while one with whole milk might have 200. Go for the skim version (enjoy the calcium boost), couple it with about 10 nuts, and call it a complete snack!

One word of warning for women: At this point, the evidence still suggests that too much caffeine may be linked to a higher rate of miscarriage. So if you're pregnant or thinking of having a baby, discuss caffeine intake with your obstetrician. In general, cutting down is a good idea.

Also, be aware that coffee isn't the only source of caffeine. A few others are listed below. Try swapping your afternoon cup for a high ORAC cup of tea. Keep in mind that the amount of caffeine listed below is just a guideline. The actual amount varies depending on brand and preparation.

Source	Serving	Caffeine
Brewed/drip coffee	6 oz	100 mg
Espresso	1 oz	40 mg
Tea (all varieties, including black, green, and white)	6 oz	40 mg
Caffeinated soft drinks	12 oz	40 mg
Hot cocoa	6 oz	7 mg

Leafy greens One study found that women who ate the most leafy green and cruciferous vegetables had brains that were 1 to 2 years "younger" in performance than those who ate fewer.[15] Smart girls eat greens? Or girls who eat greens are smart? Either way—eat up! A serving of lettuce has about 300 ORAC points.

Nutmeg While this spice that makes most of us reminisce about apple pie has been studied for its effects on blood pressure and cholesterol levels, and researchers have found it effective against bacteria such as *E. coli,* it also has a well-deserved reputation as a home remedy for anxiety: Use just a pinch in a glass of warm skim milk or orange juice and see if you don't feel better!

Oatmeal Talk about brain food! A complex carbohydrate, oatmeal causes your brain to produce serotonin, a feel-good chemical. Not only does serotonin have antioxidant properties, but it creates a soothing feeling that helps overcome stress. Studies have shown that kids who eat oatmeal for breakfast, with about 600 ORAC points per serving, stay sharper throughout the morning.[16]

Oranges I like to toss a piece of this fruit in my work bag, because oranges are as powerful as they are portable. One study found that when people are consuming plenty of vitamin C, their blood pressure and cortisol levels return to normal faster after a stressful event.[17] A medium-size navel orange has 3,000 ORAC points.

Plums These tiny treats decrease anxiety-related behaviors, and researchers think they might target the oxidative stress linked to depression. A serving of one plum adds 4,100 ORAC points to a meal.

Turmeric The bright orange spice that helps give curry its flavor contains an antioxidant called curcumin, a substance that has reduced the kinds of plaque found in Alzheimer's disease, and researchers think it may explain why so few people from India develop this tragic condition.[18] When cooking with turmeric, always add a dash of pepper—that can increase your body's ability to soak up the curcumin. The amount used in most recipes adds 3,500 ORAC points.

Walnuts Here I go again—I'm admittedly a little nuts about nuts. While many nuts are good sources of vitamin E, walnuts are extra helpful for staying sharp. They contain alpha-linolenic acid, an essential omega-3 fatty acid, and other polyphenols that have been shown to be protective against memory loss. Researchers at Tufts University found that animals that ingested walnuts even *reversed* some signs of brain aging. A serving (about seven halves) contains 1,900 ORAC points.

3

Sleep, Exercise, Stress, Your Environment, and Sex:

Five Big Fat Reasons We Struggle with Our Weight

When it comes to measuring your progress on the O₂ Diet, I'm predicting you'll lose about 2 to 3 pounds per week. But would you be stunned if I told you there are a handful of other numbers that actually matter as much—if not more—for the next 32 days? For one thing, I want you to keep as close an eye on those ORAC points, striving to consume 50,000 a day during the 4-day cleansing phase, and then at least 30,000 daily for the next 4 weeks.

Just as important, I want you to pay close attention to how many hours you sleep, how much exercise you get, and even how many times you have sex.

You heard me. Right now, how much you weigh isn't that important. You're probably thinking, *Huh? This is a* diet *book—I'm only reading it because I want to lose weight!* But I'm asking you to make a big psychological change here, and it's crucial to understand that these other numbers not only have a big impact on your weight, they are important barometers of your overall health.

When clients come to see me, it's almost always because they want to lose weight. And that makes sense. And the latest data on overweight and obesity show the problem continues to get worse.[1] It's a tremendous public health problem, costing billions in additional health care bills. On a one-on-one basis, working with clients, I get a constant close-up of the frustration, emotional pain, and genuine unhappiness that plague so many people about their weight. I can report that the pain can be just as intense for someone struggling to lose 5 pounds as for someone looking to lose 105 pounds—for most people, body weight and body image are intensely personal, emotional issues.

But weight is also a public problem. The latest numbers show that about 33 percent of American adults are overweight, which means that their body mass index (BMI), a number most experts think is more meaningful than just weight, is from 25 to 29.9. Another 33 percent of Americans are obese, which means their BMI is 30 or greater. A recent Harris poll found that 64 percent of Americans are unhappy with their weight at any given moment and that 77 percent say they have tried to lose weight in the past.[2]

On the surface, those numbers make perfect sense. It's probably the heavier people who are looking to slim down, right?

Not always. I know from my practice that many overweight people don't realize how big a problem they have, and many people with a BMI in the healthy range are tremendously unhappy with their bodies. If you've never calculated your BMI, check out the chart on page 36. Some overweight people are just in denial—their weight has been creeping up slowly, maybe only a few pounds a year. And it's not entirely their fault—because being overweight has become so common, our views have become distorted. When we see someone who is 10 or 15 pounds overweight, we just think of them as a little heavy, not exactly "fat." We certainly don't see them as clinically fat.

Body Mass Index

Look for your height in inches on the left side of the chart, then look to the right to find your weight. You'll discover your Body Mass Index at the very top of that column. Note that the BMI is just a rough estimate. Having more muscle on your frame will likely skew your BMI results, elevating you into the overweight or even obese zone when you may be perfectly normal. You can get a more accurate measure of body fatness by asking a registered dietician or trainer at your gym to give you a skin-fold thickness check with calipers.

BMI	21	22	23	24	25	26	27	28	29	30	35	40	41	42
Height (in.)	Weight (lb.)													
58	100	105	110	115	119	124	129	134	138	143	167	191	196	201
59	104	109	114	119	124	128	133	138	143	148	173	198	203	208
60	107	112	118	123	128	133	138	143	148	153	179	204	209	215
61	111	116	122	127	132	137	143	148	153	158	185	211	217	222
62	115	120	126	131	136	142	147	153	158	164	191	218	224	229
63	118	124	130	135	141	146	152	158	163	169	197	225	231	237
64	122	128	134	140	145	151	157	163	169	174	204	232	238	244
65	126	132	138	144	150	156	162	168	174	180	210	240	246	252
66	130	136	142	148	155	161	167	173	179	186	216	247	253	260
67	134	140	146	153	159	166	172	178	185	191	223	255	261	268
68	138	144	151	158	164	171	177	184	190	197	230	262	269	276
69	142	149	155	162	169	176	182	189	196	203	236	270	277	284
70	146	153	160	167	174	181	188	195	202	207	243	278	285	292
71	150	157	165	172	179	186	193	200	208	215	250	286	293	301
72	154	162	169	177	184	191	199	206	213	221	258	294	302	309
73	159	166	174	182	189	197	204	212	219	227	265	302	310	318
74	163	171	179	186	194	202	210	218	225	233	272	311	319	326
75	168	176	184	192	200	208	216	224	232	240	279	319	327	335
76	172	180	189	197	205	213	221	230	238	246	287	328	336	344

BMI CHART KEY: Normal: *18–24* **Overweight:** *25–29* **Obese:** *30–39* **Extremely obese:** *40 and above. Find an expanded BMI table at www.nhlbi.nih.gov/guidelines/obesity/bmi_tbl.pdf.*

Even doctors have gotten a distorted perspective: Only 12 percent of the population has ever been told by a doctor that they have a weight problem, according to that Harris poll. And sadly, many obese people— even some who are extremely so, and therefore at significantly higher risk for many health problems—often believe they are merely overweight. (BMI—like any other scale—is just numbers. There are incredibly fit people with high BMIs who are not *fat*. Basketball legend Shaquille O'Neal, for example, is technically obese—as are about half the members of the National Football League. And they're some of the fittest athletes ever!)

Then there are the many people with BMIs in the healthy range of 19.5 to 25 but who just don't like the way they look and are constantly trying to lose weight. To a degree, I'm all for self-improvement—if you're 5 feet 2 inches and think you would look and feel better at 105 pounds instead of 120, go for it. Both are healthy weights, so to an extent, it's just a matter of what's normal for *you*. I always ask my clients, "What is

---

Your O$_2$ Rx:

Turbocharge your weight loss

I'm so sure that keeping track of these areas will speed your weight loss that I will be asking you to record sleep, exercise, and pampering in a food journal. Find Your O$_2$ Life Journal on page 204 or download it at www.theO2diet.com.

If you want to turbocharge your weight loss, consistency is key. For the next 32 days, I want you to commit to the following steps:

- I will strive to go to bed 20 minutes earlier every night, turning the lights out by _____ p.m.
- I will remove _____ from the bedroom to limit distractions.
- I will try to spend 60 minutes more per week being active, by doing the following: _____.
- I will _____ to make my home environment healthier, more soothing, and less cluttered.
- I will try to spend 15 minutes more a day with my spouse, love interest, good friends, or family.

your normal weight?" I do this to get a sense of what's realistic for that individual. I stress that that is a very different exercise than selecting your dream weight or recounting what you weighed on your prom night or wedding day.

Unfortunately, many people cling to the idea of some unrealistic body weight, and that number comes to represent fulfillment. "If I could only lose 10 pounds," they'll tell me, "then I'll be happy." Obsessing over a number is counterproductive, and it ignores the big picture! It's important to focus on the many positive things you do on a regular basis to be healthy and feel good.

My goal is to help you realize that while, yes, what you eat determines how much you weigh, the scale is just one small part of the story. Instead, you need to recognize that in your total well-being, your BMI is just one slice of the pie (or whole grain bread). Once you begin to focus on eating well, including plenty of foods that are truly good for you, you'll start to love how healthy you feel in every other area of your life. What's the best body weight for you? Trust me, once you stop making that one number the be-all and end-all, your weight will just fall into place.

You don't believe me, do you? If you are a career dieter, someone who has been on a decades-long crusade to diet your way back into the jeans you wore in college, what I'm suggesting sounds a little too much like . . . surrender. You're afraid I may be asking you to give up on your weight-loss goals and to accept a body weight you don't like. I'm not, I promise: If you want to lose weight, I want to help you (as long as it's within the bounds of healthy guidelines). But what I *am* asking you to do is shift your focus. For the next 32 days, I want you to try to stop thinking of weight loss as a goal or a prize and just accept it as a natural by-product of following the O_2 Diet. (And I do want you to weigh yourself at least once a week while following the plan, so that if you're not losing weight fast enough—or you're losing too fast—you can make adjustments.)

It seems like a subtle difference, but it's really a major shift in thinking: There's eating right to lose weight, which you and I both know hasn't worked for you in the past—at least not for any length of time.

And then there's what I'm asking you to do right now—eating right to feel great, which will melt the weight away.

Enough about weight already! Now let's focus on some other numbers that have more impact on your weight than you probably realize.

sleep

Once upon a time, in the land before TiVo, people never worried about getting enough sleep. The sun set, it got dark, and they went to bed—there was nothing else to do. When the sun came up, they went to work again. But ever since the advent of artificial light, we've been in trouble. Today, between laptops and TV, we can keep busy 24/7. In fact, some of us have forgotten that at some point, the workday is *supposed* to end, and we even sleep with our BlackBerrys right next to us. I've been known to do this myself sometimes.

But it's making us gain weight! Experts estimate that compared to getting 7 to 8 hours per night, the risk of developing obesity rises 23 percent with just 6 hours of sleep per night, 50 percent with only 5 hours per night, and 73 percent with 4 hours per night.

We're busy people. The truth is, I have plenty of days when I think my life would be much easier if I didn't need to log hours of z's every night. But sleep is one of the most powerful antioxidant tools we have. During sleep, our body actually removes free radicals that build during waking hours. Essentially, sleep—governed by melatonin, a hormone that is one of the body's most powerful antioxidants—provides the body with a

Your O_2 Injection:
Make a sleep date

Pull out your schedule and look at your plans for the weekend: What can you cancel or reschedule to find an extra hour to do nothing but sleep? Or go ahead and enter NAP in capital letters, so you won't forget. Remember, sleep isn't for lazy people—it's a powerful antioxidant boost for your overworked brain.

natural way to repair oxidative damage. Canadian researchers think that it works like this: When we sleep, we give the cortical circuits in the brain a break, allowing them to restructure, remodel, and rebuild as the brain releases its own antioxidant chemicals to wash through the brain. If you don't sleep, your brain can't mop up the free radicals created by the stresses and strains of your busy day.[3]

If we could measure sleep in a test tube (the way foods are measured for their ORAC values), it would rate high on the ORAC scale. It's ironic—sleep is so good for us, it feels great, and it's free. You'd think people would think of it as a wonder drug and pounce on it, wouldn't you? I believe most of us *want* to sleep more; sometimes, friends and clients will tell me, "I feel like pulling out my hair—I just want to sleep!" It's just that we've forgotten how to make time for enough rest. And me? I feel like I can conquer the world on a good night's sleep. Otherwise, I'm just plain scary to be around.

Still, most of us fight sleep. While 8 hours a night is the recommended average (some people can get by on less, and there may be health risks associated with sleeping too much), the average person gets 6.9 hours per night, according to the National Sleep Foundation—6.8 hours during the week and 7.4 hours on weekends. That means that over the course of a year, the average person builds up a sleep debt of about 402 hours—we'd need to sleep 16 days straight each year to make that up! And that's just in a year. Now imagine the way you've been cheating your body of one of its best natural antioxidants over the past decade or so. In terms of sleep debt, we're seriously broke.

And we're paying the price. Today, about 56 percent of Americans say that daytime drowsiness is a problem, and 34 percent say they are sometimes dangerously sleepy;[4] drowsy driving causes about 4 percent of all car crashes. Too little sleep slows the rate at which our wounds can heal. It weakens our immune system, so we get sick more often. And as researchers become more sophisticated in their ability to measure oxidative damage, they've learned that too little sleep contributes to aging and other diseases, including heart disease.[5] Lack of sleep can also make you hungrier and crave the worst types of food.

The best solution, experts say, is to brush up on "sleep hygiene" basics.

- Set a specific bedtime.

- Put all the electronics—your TV, your computer, and, yes, even your BlackBerry—in another room.

- Start winding down about a half hour before you plan to turn in, shutting off your TV and computer. I know, it's hard to do— I can always think of one more e-mail to send before bedtime, too. But your body needs a little time to wind down before drifting off to sleep.

- Read a little, meditate, take a warm bath, listen to relaxing music, or fix a cup of herbal tea—all have been shown to help you relax.

- No more hitting the snooze button—get up when the alarm goes off! (One of my clients says she doesn't have time for the gym, but she hits snooze for 45 minutes each morning. Why hit snooze when you can sleep? I suggested she set the alarm for 45 minutes *later* most days, so she can catch up on her sleep, but get up right away on those other 3 days and finally use the elliptical that's in her basement. It's working!) The idea is to train yourself to get more deep, restorative sleep by maximizing your hours.

The good news is that once you make getting out of sleep debt a priority, you'll be amazed at how good you feel. Seriously. A leading Stanford University sleep researcher uses just one word to describe how people feel when they really and truly catch up on their sleep: *superhuman*.

As your body begins to benefit from the increased surge of antioxidants that come with enough z's, you'll feel the positive effect in every area. It's a lot easier to get excited about exercise when you're not exhausted. And when you're genuinely well rested, you don't need that 4:00 p.m. pick-me-up bag of M&Ms. You feel empowered making the right decisions about food, work, and everything else in your life.

exercise

Researchers are learning that exercise doesn't just help you lose weight, it's actually more important to your overall health than weight control is. In the "fit versus fat" debate, scientists at the University of South Carolina have shown that even obese people who exercise regularly—and I'm talking simple walking here, nothing elaborate—are healthier than normal-weight people who never break a sweat. They live longer, feel better, and are less likely to suffer from serious health problems.[6]

Of course, exercise is vital to anyone who wants to lose weight and get healthier—burning those calories will help the weight come off faster. No matter what your weight or current fitness level, several hours of exercise per week lowers your risk for heart disease, boosts bone health, and makes chronic problems like diabetes, asthma, and high blood pressure more manageable. (In some cases, exercise alone can make people healthy enough that they don't need as much—and sometimes even any—medication.) Studies have even shown exercise to be a powerful tool for fighting depression. It's perhaps the single most proven way to manage stress (I save a lot of money on therapy because I run!), and people with a moderate exercise routine also sleep better, which means they get the additional antioxidant benefit of better rest on top of the perks of working out. In terms of getting older, staying active is the best way doctors know to age gracefully. Older people who are more active get sick less often, fall less frequently, and may be less likely to develop problems like Alzheimer's disease.

Even though exercise and activity are vital to repair oxidative damage, there's a bit of a paradox: Exercise, which works by causing the body to overcome stress, actually creates free radicals. And yes, it is true—the more we exercise, the more free radicals we create. If the number of free radicals created by our workout exceeds our body's antioxidant capacity that day, those rogue molecules will harm the lipids, proteins, and DNA we need for optimal health.

As long as we're consuming enough antioxidants, exercise is amazingly good for us. Of course, we know that effect isn't just good for our hearts and other internal organs. Exercise also boosts our physical appearance by toning muscles and delivering nutrients to the skin and encouraging our bodies to carry off the toxins more efficiently—that's why exercise gives you such a gorgeous glow!

Exercise is so good for you, in fact, that it always surprises me that many people just don't like it. But it's true: The US surgeon general says about 60 percent of Americans don't get enough regular physical activity and 25 percent don't get any activity *at all*.[7]

So while all levels of moderate exercise are good, exercise combined with an antioxidant-rich plan like the O$_2$ Diet is even better. Italian researchers measured the oxidative damage in the plasma of two groups of runners. After a 60-minute run, those who had consumed higher levels of antioxidants (in this case, researchers gave them more lycopene, which is found in tomatoes and watermelon, and isoflavones, found in soy products) had much healthier levels than those who didn't have the antioxidants.[8]

If you're already a faithful exerciser, *high five to you!* I hope you'll find that following the O$_2$ Diet will give you more energy to pursue your fitness passions and maybe even the extra zip to try something new. You may think you're not bored with that same power walk every morning, but your body is—doing the same workout week after week is like constantly watching the same movie. Your body needs novel exercises to challenge it. Look for ways to throw something new into the mix to increase your fitness level instead of simply maintaining it.

- Dabble in a new type of exercise—maybe that really tough-looking balance class offered at your gym, for example. Or go for a splash in a kayak.

- At least once this week, do something that isn't your favorite so you become a more balanced athlete. If you're a devoted runner, challenge yourself to take a Pilates class. If you lift weights at the gym four times a week, plan a weekend hike with friends. If you took a Spin class yesterday, why not swim today?

- Alternate workouts. This lets all the great antioxidants you've been eating on the O$_2$ Diet go to work. In the same way that weight lifters know they need to take a day to let specific muscle groups repair (which is why they often do upper body one day and lower body the next, for example), switching activities allows those muscles and joints to rest and rebuild, too.

Your O$_2$ Breakthrough:
How hard are you working?

For some people, figuring out how intensely to exercise is baffling. I've seen people push themselves way too far early on, and others barely break a sweat. If you're not sure, here are three good ways to measure your intensity.

- **The talk test.** If you can easily sing or carry on a conversation while exercising, you probably need to step up the pace a bit. But if you're gasping out one word at a time, whoa! You're working way too hard.

- **The Centers for Disease Control and Prevention** suggests using the Borg Rating of Perceived Exertion Scale, which you'll find hanging on the walls of many gyms. It works like this: While you're working out, ask yourself how hard you're exerting yourself, and assign it a number; 6 means "no exertion at all," and 20 means "maximal exertion." This will give you a good idea of the intensity level of your activity, and you can use this information to determine how much to speed up or slow down.

6	No exertion at all
7	Extremely light
8	
9	Very light
10	
11	Light
12	
13	Somewhat hard
14	
15	Hard (heavy)
16	
17	Very hard
18	
19	Extremely hard
20	Maximal exertion

A rating of 9 corresponds to "very light" exercise. For a healthy person, that typically means walking slowly. A 13 on the scale is "somewhat hard" exercise, but it still feels okay to continue. At 17, "very hard," a healthy person can still go on but really has to push—you'll probably feel very heavy or tired.

- If you're a gadget lover, buy or borrow a heart rate monitor. Using a chest band and a wrist device, these gizmos will let you know precisely how hard you're working and give you plenty of warning when you're in or out of your target heart rate zone.

- Add interval training to your cardio routine. An easy add-in for walkers, runners, or bikers: On your usual route, pick up the pace for 30 seconds, then drop back down to normal for at least a minute to let your heart rate recover. When working out on treadmills or other machines, use the timer to add intervals, or (the easiest method) make every third song on your iPod a high-energy tune. Then push yourself again. Studies have shown that your body will continue to burn more calories for 24 hours after an interval work-out[9] and will build increased stamina. So far, researchers say, this is the best way to reduce the risk of developing diabetes.[10] (Not sure how hard you're working? Check out the chart on the opposite page.)

If you're a sporadic exerciser, I'd like you to spend a few minutes thinking about what has gotten in your way in the past. (You know better than I do how hard it is to get on track, and you have a good sense of what derails you.) I'm betting your answer is all about scheduling—work and other obligations take over the day; before you know it, even though you had the best of intentions and probably even packed your gym bag in the morning, it's 8:00 p.m. and you're exhausted. Something always comes up. And then, since you've let a week go by without a workout, you lose your motivation altogether. Since you basically have to start from scratch anyway, you figure, what's the rush?

For the next 32 days, let's try to make a plan that gets around your schedule.

- For many people, the solution is morning workouts. That way, you can cross exercise off your list *before* the crisis du jour lands on your desk.

- Put exercise in your calendar like doctor appointments, written down, so you'll be less tempted to skip it.

- Get a workout buddy and push each other! You have heard it before, but this strategy works.

- Consider hiring a personal trainer. No, I'm not saying this is a long-term solution, because it is pricey—but these days, many trainers are more flexible about their rates, and you can also share sessions with a friend or two to split costs.

- Break up exercise into minichunks. As far as your heart rate—and your body's antioxidative mechanisms—is concerned, three 10-minute walks are just as beneficial as a 30-minute one.

- Strive for consistency, with three times a week as your starting goal.

- Be honest about boredom. It's hard to do something faithfully if it doesn't appeal to you—so what *do* you like to do? If you've joined and unjoined a number of gyms, I think we can safely say, "Wake up—you're not a gym person!" Are you, perhaps, a dance person? If so, find a local ballroom studio and commit to a series of classes. Always had a fantasy about learning to figure skate or mastering a martial art? Sign up! For people like you, fitness isn't about finding discipline, it's about finding *fun*.

If you just don't like to exercise, you're one of a large group of people—about 25 percent. Believe me, I'm sympathetic. Personally, I have always liked working out. I love sports and am crazy about lifting weights—although I'll admit that sometimes my "weight training" occurs not at the gym but at home, lifting my 3-year-old. And I have a great time (and a terrific workout) chasing after my kids. But in my nutrition practice, I've come to understand how many people just loathe exercise—they don't like to sweat, they'd rather wear high heels than sneakers, and the very idea of working that hard makes them head for the couch.

I have good news: The most recent federal guidelines have made your life easier. Instead of recommending exercise in sweaty 30-minute blocks, they now use the gentler "activity" phrase. No gym required!

- Clean the house. Hey, somebody has to do it. And yes, it burns calories! Dusting, vacuuming, and mopping all count.

- Shop. Take 2 extra laps around the sale racks at Bloomingdale's, or march up and down the mall a time or two.

- Watch the clock. My plea is that for the next 32 days, as you follow the O$_2$ Diet, you try to be active for 2½ hours a week, mixing up your activities to keep it interesting. Aim for at least 10 minutes a day.

- Think about something you've never tried before, like a yoga or tai chi class. Not only do both have proven stress-reduction (and antioxidant-boosting) powers, they often appeal to people who don't think of themselves as athletic. Ballet for grown-ups or African dance classes, which often incorporate beautiful music into classes, also have devoted followings. Willing to give something like that a try?

If you're an intense exerciser and weekend warrior, by now you've noticed that I keep saying "moderate exercise." In fact, because I'm guessing you're a type A personality like me, the phrase *moderate exercise* is probably getting on your nerves. But I use that term deliberately. Intense exercise increases oxidative damage and in many ways harms the body's ability to fend off free radicals. Does that mean I expect you to abandon your plans to climb Kilimanjaro or cycle cross-country? No way! The more I sweat, the better I feel. In college, I was a lacrosse player. I've done the New York City Marathon, and I'm a triathlete. I get it! Over the years, I've worked with professional athletes, too, helping them come up with nutrition plans that enable them to train intensely.

But I'd be lying if I didn't acknowledge that our bodies pay a cellular price for that level of intensity. In a perfect world, there would be no need to worry: A Japanese study that measured oxidative damage in runners in a 2-day ultramarathon—could you get any more extreme?—found that levels of oxidative stress in the runners' plasma began returning to normal when the race was over.[11] But because type A people tend to neglect themselves in other ways—overtraining even when we know better—intense exercise can be more of a health risk than a health benefit. For example, the body's natural killer cells (vital to our immune function) increase in activity after a moderate workout or very short burst of intense exercise. But they actually decline after workouts that are too long or too hard.[12] And studies have shown that while people who work out moderately, in 40-minute sessions, get about half as many colds as the average person, intense workouts of 90 minutes—like long training runs—actually weaken your immune system, putting you at risk for getting sick for a full 72 hours after each workout.[13] That means you have to make other changes in your lifestyle, including diet, sleep, and stress management, to allow your body to offset those tougher workouts.

So 2 days a week, timed to your toughest workouts:

- Increase your antioxidant intake to 50,000 points.
- Get an extra half hour of sleep.
- Make a small part of the workout, maybe the cooldown or stretch, be all about relaxation, not exertion.

Whatever type of exercise you are doing, be consistent. Put it in the book and stick to it!

stress (and destressing)

We all have stress in our daily lives. To a degree, it's perfectly healthy. It's how we're designed: Back in those pre-TiVo days, we'd be faced with a hostile woolly mammoth or saber-toothed tiger, and our body would respond by instantly switching to fight-or-flight mode, producing a high-octane combination of chemicals like adrenaline, cortisol, epinephrine, and norepinephrine. We'd escape, the danger would pass, and our body would cheerfully reabsorb those chemicals—and we'd reward ourselves with a big handful of healthy, antioxidant-laden berries and a long nap.

But the problem is that for many of us, stress has become a semipermanent state, with woolly mammoths lurking around every corner. These days, they take the shape of work deadlines, family pressures, financial worries, too little sleep, or even wonderful things like a new baby. We're so used to living with the symptoms of chronic stress—forgetfulness, irritability, anxiety, depression—that we barely notice them. We start to think that's who we are.

Our bodies never get the chance to process those stress chemicals, and they're in our blood far too often. It's this chemical cascade that has been proven to create severe oxidative damage and is known to cause heart disease, high blood pressure, and stroke. It's also strongly linked to cancer, diabetes, and depression.

Excess stress also creates lots of little health problems that may not kill us but certainly keep us from feeling our best. These include digestive problems, heart palpitations, headaches, menstrual issues, pain, fatigue, cold sores, skin problems, and even allergies.

Stress saps our bodies' strength and weakens their ability to do what they're supposed to. Almost instinctively, we know we can combat this with the foods we eat. For example, all carbohydrates signal the brain to make more serotonin, a feel-good brain chemical that has an antioxidative effect and can combat the free radicals generated by all that surging cortisol. (See—you knew there was a reason you craved those high-carb baked goods during stressfests!) But eating the wrong carbs (or just overeating, perhaps because you're worried or stressed about something) sets you up for a crash in a few hours. On the O_2 Diet, I suggest you eat plenty of wholesome whole grains—high-fiber whole wheat bread products, oatmeal, and quinoa. Because whole grains are digested more slowly, they release a steadier stream of serotonin and keep your blood sugar more stable.

Here's your plan to relieve stress:

- Spend 5 minutes "stressing." Giving yourself a little time to get all the worrying out of your system will enable you to let go for a bit for the rest of the day.

- Ditch your cell for at least an hour a day. Cutting down on multitasking—and the need to feel like you're always "on"—will make you feel calmer.

- Take a mindful minute. Mindfulness—the term stress experts use for being fully aware of what we're doing at exactly that moment, whether it's eating a raspberry or listening to a friend—is deeply restorative. It's also hard to do; most of us tend to have our minds going a mile a minute. Set aside some time each day to really be fully present.

- Go to the park. A recent University of Michigan study found that people who spent an hour walking in the park lowered their stress levels and improved their capacity to pay attention, compared to people who spent an hour walking through town.[14] Trees are soothing!

- Pamper yourself! Not only is taking care of yourself good for relieving stress, but sometimes how we take care of ourselves can actually benefit our inner stress levels *and* outer beauty. We will get to much more on this topic in Chapter 6, but for now, take some time to bathe, scrub, moisturize, or get a massage. Or all of the above!

environment

When it comes to wreaking oxidative damage, environmental factors are huge. Air pollution, noise pollution, light pollution, and electromagnetic risks all take their toll, causing our bodies to generate free radicals much faster than if we lived in pristine, remote mountain areas.

Researchers have linked many types of pollution with cancer and other diseases—and it's not just the junk we breathe. Noise pollution wears us out, too: Studies have shown that people who live closer to airports have significantly elevated levels of cortisol, the stress hormone, than people who live in quieter areas.[15] And light pollution has been linked to cancer.

Yet in some ways, for all the talk about global warming and the efforts to take better care of the planet, it's hard for many of us to think about the toll our environment takes on our personal health. Part of it is that on an individual basis, we're pretty powerless. We can't order the East Coast to turn off its lights, single-handedly repair the ozone layer, or even do much to control traffic noise in our own neighborhoods. And

Your O$_2$ Injection:

Make your air greener

A pretty way to clean the air you breathe is to add plants to your home and office: A NASA study looked at the ability of 19 common houseplants to purify the air and found that philodendrons, English ivy, and spider plants were among the best performers.[16] Bonus: They're among the easiest to grow!

for most of us, leaving isn't an option, either—between work, friends, and family, we are attached to where we live.

But that doesn't mean we can't take steps to improve our home environments. One of the easiest things to do is streamline a little—clutter causes stress. (Don't you hate the anxiety that comes from storming around trying to find your keys?)

We can eliminate toxic cleaning products. As much as I love to use vinegars in food, because—you guessed it—varieties like apple cider and red wine vinegar are powerful antioxidants, white vinegar cleans an amazing number of surfaces without generating any damaging fumes. And there are plenty of chemical-free products you can buy, too.

Again, let me reassure you that eating well, including an antioxidant-rich diet, does protect you. Researchers at the National Institutes of Health have found that people who consume more antioxidants are better able to shake off the damaging effects of smog.[17]

To protect your environment:

- Make some corner of your life—your desk, your bedroom, or even your car—a clutter-free zone.

- Cut down on noise by closing windows. Turn off the TV when you aren't really watching.

sex

Sex is a silent casualty of our too-busy lifestyle. It's the subject of just about every sitcom, so you'd think we were a very sexually active society. But in my practice, I constantly see people for whom sex is a problem—they're tired, their libido is low, and their spouse may even be complaining of neglect. (Some studies have shown that as many as 33 percent of all women and, despite all the stereotypes, as many as 20 percent of men suffer from low libido at some point.)[18] Don't think my husband hasn't heard me snap, "Because I'm tired—that's why!" more than a few times.

Is there a link between low libido and weight? Absolutely! Up to 30 percent of people who struggle with their weight also report problems with sex drive, desire, or performance, according to researchers at Duke University.[19] As many 50 percent of all people with diabetes, many of whom are also overweight, complain of some level of sexual dysfunction.[20]

Certainly, some of the connection is about self-esteem and body image. But some of it is physiological: The more body fat you have, the more it secretes sex hormone binding globulin, or SBGH, which binds to testosterone, the sex hormone found in both men and women. Researchers believe that too much SBGH means there is less free testosterone to stimulate libido.[21] Losing as little as 10 pounds is enough to increase sex drive, they've discovered.

The good news is that not only does losing weight help your sex life, but having sex also helps your weight loss! First of all, while it's not (usually!) as strenuous as an afternoon of tennis, sex does burn calories. Second, researchers know that oxytocin—a hormone secreted in the neurons of the pituitary gland and released in both men and women after orgasm, through cuddling, and even by simply holding hands—acts as a soothing antioxidant[22] and may make it easier for people to stick to their diets.[23]

Oxytocin makes us healthier in other ways. For years, scientists have known that this hormone, sometimes called the "calm and connection hormone," does a lot. For example, in women, it signals when to go into labor and controls milk flow during breastfeeding. It's also key in establishing maternal behavior and in how much we trust people. How powerful is it? A University of North Carolina study found that when couples spent just 10 minutes holding hands, oxytocin levels rose enough to significantly lower blood pressure.[24] And since women who breastfeed have lower risks of breast cancer, heart disease, stroke, high blood pressure, and diabetes, some researchers believe that elevated levels of oxytocin may be part of the explanation, offering protection.[25]

Sex and cuddling aren't the only ways to generate this feel-good antioxidant. Spending time with animals is beneficial—some studies have found that people generate more oxytocin spending time with their pets than with their spouse! And hugs from friends and family help, too.

To me, how much time you spend with the people you love isn't important just from a chemical perspective. (But admit it—isn't it cool to know that something that feels as good as sex is also really good for you?) It's about living a balanced life. When I hear a client talking about spending more time with her spouse—whether it's having sex or going to the movies—it makes me happy. I know the switch has been flipped, and that she is getting the idea that she can restore balance to her busy life. Investing time in our relationships is just as important as wrapping up that report by deadline, making it to the gym, or eating well—it's one more way we say, "I deserve to have a nutritious life—good for me on every level."

4

The O$_2$ Diet's 32-Day Plan:

Eat More (ORAC), Feel Great, Look Fantastic

You now know the science behind why antioxidants are so good for you. And you know how they will help everything from your skin to your heart to your waistline. But what exactly are you supposed to eat? How much? And when? That is what this chapter is all about.

The O$_2$ Diet involves four distinctly different phases, each designed to flow one right after the other, each carefully controlled for the right number of antioxidants and portions.

O$_2$ Phase I You'll start here, with the 4-Day O$_2$ Cleanse. This intense phase is slightly lower in calories than the rest of the plan so that you maximize your initial weight loss. Most people will lose about 2 to 5 pounds in this period, and that early success is important both physically and psychologically. But Phase I is also *much* higher in antioxidants— 50,000 points per day—so you'll benefit from the feel-good power of these antioxidants almost immediately.

O$_2$ Phase II This 2-week phase will provide at least 30,000 ORAC points per day. Remember, a high-ORAC plan is important because the more points you consume, the better your body will be able to mop up the free radicals in your bloodstream and the better you'll look and feel.

The portions, and thus the calories, are clearly spelled out (allowing you to adjust for your own weight), making this the part of the O₂ Diet in which you'll lose the most weight and your body will become accustomed to consuming much more fresh food than you have in the past. Trust me, by the end of these 2 weeks, you'll not only be thinner, but you'll also be craving your fruits and veggies! (I've also given you a do-it-yourself plan, so you can incorporate the foods you love most.)

O₂ Phase III The next 2-week phase is nothing complicated. It's basically the same as Phase II, except you add *conscious indulgences* as well as a few more food options. You will still track your ORAC points to make sure you eat at least 30,000 a day, and you'll continue to lose weight, but at a slightly slower pace than in the early weeks on the plan. There's real science behind this strategy: Those little extras will make it more likely that you'll continue this new, healthy eating model until you reach your weight-loss goals and beyond. Phase III allows for more real-life options—such as how to eat at restaurants and when you are on the go.

O₂ for Life! By this phase, you will have become so used to this style of eating that anything fewer than 30,000 ORAC points—which usually

---

Your O₂ Breakthrough:

O₂ and portion size

I'm sure you've seen all the news reports saying that portion control is, well, out of control! How can we get it reined in without carrying around a food scale? On the O₂ Diet, your focus is on putting the most nutrient-dense foods into your body. But there still have to be limits—I get a lot of people in my office who are overweight from eating way too many *healthy* foods!

I'll get into specifics about portion size later in the chapter. For now, keep in mind that when it comes to veggies, you can go crazy! I want you to use veggies to fill up. This is why I don't give portions for veggies in the 4-day cleanse or the 2-week plan. One caveat: If those veggies have added fat, stick to the portions in the chart and do *not* feel free to "eat as much as you want." Otherwise, the portions listed in the veggie section are the *minimum* I want you to have. Feel free to double veggie portions at lunch and dinner especially. I have never had a client not lose weight because she ate 1½ cups of spinach!

translates into anywhere between five and nine generous produce servings throughout the day—will simply feel wrong for your body. You won't have to track the points—your body will tell you when it's not getting enough. But I do suggest that you keep a food journal for the long haul— you will reach your points daily if you follow the O_2 Diet guidelines, *and* you'll be more likely to maintain your weight loss when you track what you eat. Additionally, the O_2 for Life phase includes a Q&A in the back of the book that gives you even more real-world, long-term eating strategies designed to help you handle things like working late, missing a meal, or coping with the occasional overindulgence.

O_2 phase I: the 4-day O_2 cleanse

We begin with a supercharged ORAC cleanse. "Cleanse" can sound intimidating, but I wouldn't ask you to jump in if it were not for good reason. In 4 quick days, there are many benefits you will feel *and* see! Your pants may loosen up a bit. People may comment on how great your skin looks. You will have more energy. Most of all, you will gain a sense of empowerment. An "I want to put good things in my body" feeling will begin to take charge.

Why cleanse? A cleanse is a way to jump-start not only weight loss but also good behaviors. I like to look at it as the framework of the plan. You'll establish the right behaviors and eat the right foods; in the subsequent phases, you'll build on that strong foundation. A cleanse may seem daunting at first, but if you push yourself to implement these practices over the next 4 days, you will see a difference, and it will be easier to build upon your early success.

How is the cleanse different from the rest of the plan? The cleanse is slightly less caloric, has no variety, has less sodium and sugar, and is higher in ORAC points. By reducing calories a bit more dramatically over the next 4 days, you ensure that you kick-start a change in your weight, sense of well-being, and overall health.

Why no variety on the cleanse? If you follow the cleanse to the letter, I know *and* you know that you will get over 50,000 ORAC points. A little boring, I admit, but it's the easiest way to get you started without having to work *too* hard at learning points. Yes, variety is important for long-term maintenance of a diet, but in the short term *little* variety is very helpful. No choices means no options, which means no veering off track. Limiting your menu makes it easy to shop and gets you in the zone with what you should be buying at the grocery store.

No salt shaker, please! The cleanse strips your diet of much added sodium and sugar. You'll notice you are eating all whole foods. Right away this helps you shed a little water weight. How does that make you feel? You got it—excellent! So you may have a tad more breathing room in those jeans that have been hanging in the back of your closet. This cleanse will help flush you out, starting you on the right track with your weight and mind-set.

Why 50,000 ORAC points? Think of it as making up for lost time. I bet if you could calculate the ORAC points you have consumed over the past year or week, you would be falling short. Even if you like your fruits and veggies and stay away from the latest cupcake shop, you will see how easy it is to get so much ORAC in your life. The benefits will start to show right away. You will have improved energy, have shed about 2 to 5 pounds, and see an improvement in your skin—watch out, world, you may just glow! At the same time, you are setting yourself up with some excellent behaviors and the framework for a high-ORAC life.

When should you begin the cleanse? I am tempted to say "this minute." But I will try not to be overzealous. I see people putting off a cleanse until after vacation, or after a deadline, or after . . . When I hear clients utter these words, I usually respond: "It will always be someone's birthday or a 'busy' week! You need to begin living a better life *now!*" Okay, I realize not everyone is going to begin the O₂ Diet this actual minute. Here's my advice to the procrastinators in the bunch: Don't wait too long. Pick the clearest 4 days in the next week or two. *No* putting off longer than that. Make an appointment to go to the grocery store the day before you start the cleanse, schedule the 4 days of exercise, and even write in when you will pamper yourself and when you will go to bed. Finished looking at your calendar? Great! You have a date to get moving.

4-DAY O₂ CLEANSE

Follow this plan exactly for the next 4 days!

BREAKFAST

Scrambled eggs (1 whole omega-3-enriched egg plus 3 egg whites)*

1 teaspoon dried basil

1 cup green tea

1 cup water with 1 ounce lemon juice

SNACK

Sliced Granny Smith apple with 1 teaspoon cinnamon

LUNCH

Spinach (cooked or raw); eat as much spinach as you'd like. And have fun dressing the spinach with flavored vinegars, such as fig, raspberry, or orange. Any type of vinegar will do.

4 ounces salmon or halibut (grilled, baked, or broiled)* with 1 teaspoon dried spices, such as oregano

8 pecan halves

1 cup water with 1 ounce lemon juice

SNACK

Steamed artichoke or ½ cup artichoke hearts in water (Monterey Farms makes an easy eat-right-out-of-the-bag variety.)

1 cup green tea

DINNER

Large romaine lettuce salad with carrots, tomatoes, and red bell peppers; dress with 1 teaspoon extra virgin olive oil and lemon juice to taste

Steamed asparagus

4 ounces any lean protein (grilled, baked, or broiled; see the "Lean Protein" list on page 84) with spices such as 1 teaspoon oregano

1 cup water with 1 ounce lemon juice

1 cup blueberries

ORAC Value: 57,300

*If you don't like eggs or fish, feel free to substitute firm tofu and/or fresh, lean turkey.

During these 4 days, I also want you to:

DRINK

- 8 total glasses of water (Aim for each glass to include 1 ounce of lemon juice.)
- 2 cups of green tea

SLEEP (and HAVE SEX)

- Sleep 7 to 8 hours per night. This sounds simple enough, but too many of you do not do it! Make it happen at least for these 4 days.
- For all the reasons I mention in Chapter 3, try to have sex. If it doesn't happen, no big deal. Try to spend some time with friends and family.

PAMPER

- Spend a little time babying yourself; this will remind you that this plan isn't about deprivation but about treating yourself to the very best, inside and out. A little pampering aids in alleviating stress and will help you to look and feel your absolute best. Much, much more about this in Chapter 6!
- Cleanse your face twice daily (choose one treatment from the list beginning on page 149).*
- Scrub your face and body (choose one treatment from the list beginning on page 150) on day 1 and day 4.*

DESTRESS

- When you drink a cup of green tea or an extra cup of herbal tea, make sure you savor it in quiet, by yourself, taking some time alone.
- Take 15 minutes to do something just for you! And make it something you don't normally take time for, such as using that lavender bath oil that you have been saving for just the right moment.

If you don't have time to create your own treatment, using your store-bought favorite product is fine as well!.

IMPROVE YOUR ENVIRONMENT

- In Chapter 3, I asked you to do one thing to make your home environment healthier. Over the next 4 days, try to make one additional improvement to your home or make one change to another environment you frequent, such as your office.

EXERCISE

- Each day do 45 minutes of any cardio activity you love. If you haven't gotten off the couch in years, "cardio" may mean walking. For the rest of you, I want you to exercise so hard so that it's a little tough to speak in full sentences. If you can speak in a conversational tone, you're not working hard enough; if you can only get out single words, back off.

- Stretch 5 minutes in the a.m. and 5 minutes in the p.m.

O₂ CLEANSE SHOPPING LIST

Take this list with you to the store. You can also download it at www.theO2diet.com. It contains everything you need to complete the cleanse. Easy as that.

1 dozen omega-3-enriched eggs

4 Granny Smith apples

4 cups blueberries

6 (at least) lemons

16 ounces of a combination of canned salmon, fresh salmon, and halibut

16 ounces other lean protein (see the "Lean Protein" list, page 84)

4 artichokes, two 8-ounce cans artichokes (rinse under cold water to remove sodium), or 4 packages Monterey Farms ArtiHearts

Spinach

Romaine

Asparagus

Carrots

Plum tomatoes

Red bell peppers

2 ounces pecans

Cold-pressed (expeller-pressed) olive oil

Green tea

Basil, dried

Cinnamon, ground

Oregano, dried

O₂ phase II: the next 2 weeks

The easiest way to approach this phase is to simply follow the O₂ Phase II diet plan I have designed. But if you are feeling creative or are convinced you don't like some of these foods, you can skip ahead to the O₂ Do-It-Yourself Plan.

If you choose the O₂ 2-week meal plan, I've already done the math, so you don't have any homework, adding up points!

If you choose the DIY option, what's the best way to add up your points? Use the O₂ Life Journal (see page 204, or visit www.theO2diet.com to download the journal and an ORAC points portable guide). Make journaling a habit. Studies show that people who keep food journals are more likely to not only lose weight but keep the weight off for the long term. Jot down each food in your journal and simply add in your points in the next line. If writing it down is tough for you, try keeping a draft running in your BlackBerry or iPhone. If adding up points is too much for you, don't stress out. If you are choosing from the building blocks (which we will get to in a few pages), you're bound to be on track.

Either way, you'll notice that the framework is similar to the cleanse. The main differences are that you will have a lot of wonderful ORAC variety and, because you are adding in a starch serving to breakfast and having slightly bigger snacks, a slightly higher caloric range. (You'll still lose weight, I promise.) You will begin to see how you can eat this way wherever you are, feel more satisfied, and enjoy the most nutritious foods in the world—all at the same time you are continuing to slim, glow, and soar!

Snack. You must snack! You need to snack to keep your metabolism revved and to keep your hunger quotient, or HQ, in check until your next meal so you don't overdo it. (We'll talk more about HQ later in this chapter.) Snacking is an opportunity to give your body more nutrients—yes, you got it—more ORAC! A snack should be portion controlled (you only need a little fuel to keep you energized and burning calories) and provide, in addition to some ORAC, a combination of fiber, protein, and/or healthy fat to keep you satisfied. When you snack, you are less likely to overeat at the next meal and you keep your metabolism revved. Both are essential for weight loss.

O$_2$ PHASE II GUIDELINES

Whether you choose the O$_2$ Phase II 2-week meal plan I designed or the O$_2$ Phase II DIY plan, there are a few principles you must apply for this to be effective.

- Eat 30,000 (or more) ORAC points per day (within the diet guidelines).
- Begin each day with a glass of water with 1 ounce of lemon juice.
- Have at least 8 glasses of water per day, and aim to add 1 ounce of lemon juice to each glass.

Your O$_2$ Breakthrough:
You don't have to be a chef to do the O$_2$ Diet!

During the next 2 weeks, when you see a recipe and don't want to cook it, you can simply substitute a DIY meal (page 68).

For example, on Monday, instead of the Salmon with Raspberry-Balsamic Glaze, you can choose a vegetable, protein, fat, and herb or spice. Or, if you're going to a diner or your favorite Italian restaurant, order a tricolored salad and add 1 tablespoon of an oil-based dressing. Then have steamed green beans and grilled salmon. (Add black pepper to the salmon for a kick of flavor and ORAC!)

- Have at least 2 cups of green tea per day.

- Eat two snacks per day.

- Use herbs and spices as much as possible (aim for adding them to breakfast, lunch, and dinner daily).

- Use your O$_2$ Life Journal to help you keep track of your food and your ORAC points.

- Continue to aim for those 7 to 8 hours of sleep per night. Make a nap date if you fall short.

- Whatever type of exerciser you may be, be *consistent*. Put your workouts in your calendar like doctor appointments, and stick to them.

- Pamper yourself as you did during the cleanse. Hopefully, cleansing and moisturizing your skin has become a habit.

- Continue to be aware of and address your environment, sex life, and stress levels.

The O₂ 2-Week Meal Plan

If you are the type of person who likes to be told exactly what to do, then this laid-out Phase II meal plan is ideal for you. It's truly a no-brainer—just eat the foods I've listed, in the portions I've outlined. If no portions are indicated, as is the case for veggies, that

	Monday	Tuesday	Wednesday
Breakfast	1 peach ¾ c fat-free plain Greek yogurt 8 pecan halves ½ tsp cinnamon	Paradise Smoothie (pg 111)	1 slice whole grain toast ½ c fat-free cottage cheese ¼ sliced avocado ½ tsp black pepper (mix black pepper into cottage cheese, spread on toast, and top with avocado)
Snack	Celery with 2 tsp almond butter ¼ tsp cinnamon	Sliced red bell peppers 8 pecan halves	Blanched asparagus 2 Tbsp guacamole
Lunch	Quick Cobb Salad (pg 120)	Chopped romaine salad with red and yellow bell peppers, broccoli, carrots 1 c black bean soup 2 tsp olive oil (and balsamic vinegar to taste) 1 tsp cilantro (in soup)	Spinach (raw), red onion, tomato 4 oz canned salmon 2 tsp olive oil mixed with 2 Tbsp lemon juice 1 tsp pepper
Snack	¾ c fat-free plain Greek yogurt 2 oz pomegranate juice ½ c blueberries	2 figs 8 hazelnuts	Granny Smith apple 2 tsp peanut butter ¼ tsp cinnamon
Dinner	Salmon with Raspberry-Balsamic Glaze (pg 132)	Steamed asparagus 4 oz roasted chicken (no skin) 2 Tbsp Parmesan cheese (on asparagus) Tarragon (on chicken)	Sautéed kale 4 oz roasted pork tenderloin 2 tsp olive oil (on kale) Fresh sage (on pork)
TOTAL ORAC POINTS	34,700	41,600	33,300

means you can eat these foods to your HQ's content. (If you don't like the foods in this meal plan, or if you are ambitious enough to create a do-it-yourself version of this phase, skip ahead to page 68 for a plan you can customize.)

Thursday	Friday	Saturday	Sunday
Veggie and Cheddar Miniquiches (pg 109)	¾ c oat bran flakes 1 c fat-free milk 2 Tbsp ground flaxseed ½ tsp cinnamon	1 c blackberries 3 egg whites/1 yolk omelet (add mushrooms, spinach) ½ c fat-free cottage cheese (place in omelet or on side) 1 tsp basil (in omelet)	Green Tea Walnut Loaf (pg 110)
Carrots 2 tsp peanut butter ¼ tsp cinnamon	Broccoli dipped in ½ c salsa 7 walnut halves	Steamed artichoke dipped in 2 tsp olive oil mixed with 2 Tbsp lemon juice	Tomatoes 10 almonds
Steamed broccoli 4 oz white meat turkey burger 2 tsp olive oil (on broccoli) 1 tsp garlic powder (on broccoli)	Tuna and Chickpea Salad (pg 125)	Sliced tomatoes 4 oz grilled chicken 1 oz part-skim mozzarella 1 tsp basil Fig vinegar to taste	Plum and Pecan Spinach Salad with Pomegranate Dressing (pg 124)
¾ c fat-free plain Greek yogurt 2 tsp peanut butter ¼ tsp cinnamon	Celery sticks ¼ c black bean dip	1 c blueberries 8 pecan halves	¾ c cherries 10 almonds
Flank Steak with Chimichurri Sauce and Mashed Cauliflower (pg 140)	Broiled brussels sprouts 4 oz turkey burger (white meat) 2 tsp olive oil (on brussels sprouts) Pepper, basil (in turkey burger)	Spinach, Bok Choy, and Tofu Stir-Fry (pg 145)	Steamed spinach 4 oz grilled scallops 2 tsp olive oil (use to grill scallops) 1 tsp chili powder
37,500	35,100	38,900	33,300

(continued)

The O$_2$ 2-Week Meal Plan—*cont.*

	Monday	Tuesday	Wednesday
Breakfast	1 c cantaloupe $\frac{1}{2}$ c fat-free plain cottage cheese 10 almonds $\frac{1}{2}$ tsp cinnamon	1 packet plain oatmeal 1 c fat-free milk 2 Tbsp ground flaxseed $\frac{1}{2}$ tsp cinnamon	1 slice oat nut toast 1 c fat-free milk 2 tsp peanut butter (on toast) $\frac{1}{2}$ tsp cinnamon
Snack	Celery 2 Tbsp hummus $\frac{1}{4}$ tsp paprika	Sliced plum tomatoes 2 Tbsp hummus	Carrots 10 almonds
Lunch	Steamed green beans 4 oz grilled salmon 1 Tbsp chopped almonds (on green beans) 1 or 2 sprigs dill (on salmon)	Sautéed broccoli rabe 1 c black bean soup 2 tsp olive oil (on broccoli rabe) Garlic and onion powder (on soup, to taste)	Raw spinach salad with plum tomatoes and red onions 4 oz firm tofu 1 oz reduced-fat feta cheese 2 Tbsp lemon juice Salt and pepper to taste (on salad)
Snack	1 c edamame $\frac{1}{4}$ tsp black pepper and sea salt to taste	1 cup green tea with 6 oz steamed soy milk and $\frac{1}{4}$ tsp cinnamon 10 almonds	$\frac{3}{4}$ c cherries 10 almonds
Dinner	Sage-Crusted Chicken Tenders and Crispy Kale "Chips" (pg 136)	Steamed broccoli 4 oz grilled shrimp 2 tsp olive oil 1 tsp garlic and red pepper flakes to taste	Steamed artichoke 4 oz grilled chicken sausage 2 tsp olive oil mixed with 2 Tbsp lemon juice and 1 tsp garlic powder (for artichoke)
TOTAL ORAC POINTS	31,100	43,600	30,000

Thursday	Friday	Saturday	Sunday
Salmon and Feta Omelet with Asparagus (pg 108)	1 c raspberries $\frac{1}{2}$ c fat-free cottage cheese 8 pecans $\frac{1}{2}$ tsp cinnamon	$\frac{3}{4}$ c oat bran flakes 1 c fat-free milk 2 Tbsp ground flaxseed $\frac{1}{2}$ tsp cinnamon	1 c blackberries 1 c fat-free milk 2 Tbsp ground flaxseed 1 c ice $\frac{1}{2}$ tsp cinnamon (blend all for shake)
Veggie Crunch (pg 91)	Steamed artichoke dipped in 2 tsp olive oil mixed with 2 Tbsp lemon juice	Green beans 18 pistachios	Carrots 2 tsp peanut butter $\frac{1}{4}$ tsp cinnamon
Roast Beef Roll-Ups (pg 122)	Crunchy Chicken Salad Boats (pg 127)	Tuna and Chickpea Salad (pg 125)	Chopped arugula salad with tomatoes, carrots, and salsa 4 oz grilled chicken 2 Tbsp guacamole Parsley, squeeze of lime, black pepper, and sea salt (all to taste)
$\frac{3}{4}$ c fat-free plain Greek yogurt 2 oz pomegranate juice $\frac{1}{2}$ c blueberries	2 figs 8 hazelnuts	Sliced pear 1 Tbsp chopped walnuts $\frac{1}{4}$ tsp cinnamon	$\frac{3}{4}$ c fat-free plain Greek yogurt 1 c raspberries
Sesame Tuna with Jicama-Cabbage Slaw (pg 142)	Raw spinach salad, with red onions, mushrooms, tomatoes 4 oz grilled lean steak 1 Tbsp chopped walnuts Red wine vinegar Black pepper and onion powder (on steak, to taste)	Chickpea and Cauliflower Curry (pg 144)	Chili-Lime Mackerel with Mango-Avocado Salsa (pg 138)
30,200	41,600	31,100	34,900

If you don't feel like making these recipes, feel free to choose from the DIY building blocks on page 73.

the O$_2$ do-it-yourself plan

If you want to be imaginative, the DIY plan is for you. For each meal—breakfast, lunch, dinner—and snacks, choose accordingly from the lists of foods provided for each building block (food group). Use the charts that begin on page 78. You'll notice that the ORAC points are noted, and the portions are already done for you! All you need to do is choose appropriately and then add up your points.

If you're going with the DIY plan, there are a few other things you'll need to keep in mind in addition to the Phase II guidelines I offered you earlier. If you're a DIYer, you're clearly a trailblazer, so I'm confident you can absorb this extra information without getting too bogged down.

O$_2$ AND THE BALANCED PLATE

Just as we couldn't live on a fat-free diet, an all-fiber diet, or (as we certainly all know by now) an all-protein diet, we can't live on an antioxidant diet *alone* (more on this in the O$_2$ Breakthrough on page 95). Other foods and components of food are important—very important. The O$_2$ Diet will give you the right proportion of nutrients: the right ratio of carbs to fat to protein.

- Many starches and all meat, fish, milk, and yogurt are not given ORAC values. That is because their all-star nutrients are not ORAC nutrients. But that does not mean they do not have their own power-player nutrients and are not important to our diet.

- The starches I have chosen are those high in ORAC points. They are also high in fiber and low in sugar. I have included a few starches that have not been tested for an ORAC value but can boast being high in fiber, low in sugar, and packed with B vitamins.

- Protein foods (such as meat and fish) are not traditional ORAC foods, but they are essential to our diet. I have chosen some protein foods that are lean or high in omega-3s.

- The milk, yogurt, and soy products I have chosen are high in calcium and protein and lower in sugar.

- The fats I've selected include both monounsaturated and polyunsaturated fats as well as essential fatty acids (omega-3s). As much as possible, I steer clear of the saturated fats (such as those found in butter, meats, and trans fat products) that are linked to so many health problems.

- And don't forget that those ORAC foods you love have other key nutrients as well. For example, vegetables and fruits are sources of fiber.

O_2 NUTRIENT DENSITY

I use the term *nutrient density* about as often as I say, "No, you can't play any more Wii today!" *Nutrient density* is a term I simply love! It essentially encapsulates what this whole book is about. Nutrient density refers to how much meaningful value a food has. The focus of the O_2 Diet, of course, is antioxidant value, but most of the ORAC foods I list for you also are nutrient dense for other reasons. For example, the starches I list are high in fiber. Fiber helps to keep you full. Thus, these starches are more nutrient dense than fiber-free white bread. Fruits and veggies are obviously high in ORAC value but also have fiber and other vitamins, minerals, and nutrients. The milks and yogurts I recommend provide calcium with little fat and less sugar than many other sources. And, finally, the fats in the O_2 Diet are healthy fats, helping the body carry out many important functions.

O_2 AND HQ: HOW HUNGRY ARE YOU?

How hungry are you when you eat? This is one of the first questions I ask my clients. Some answer, "I eat all the time! I have no idea!" Others answer, "I wait until I am shaking, then dive into the first edible thing around!" Neither is what I want you to do. You need to become in touch with what I call your *hunger quotient* (HQ). You need to fire up your metabolism by eating breakfast every morning and then eat consistently throughout the day (this is why you will see snacks on your plan). On a scale of 1 through 10, 1 is "stuffed" and 10 is "famished." I want you to be between a 6 ("slightly hungry") and a 4 ("slightly satisfied") all the time. Your HQ will help you control portions and keep your metabolism revved. Listen to your body!

What's Your Hunger Quotient?

Hunger Quotient (HQ)	Translation
1. Stuffed (to the point of not feeling well)	I'm never eating again!
2. Extremely full	I couldn't eat another bite!
3. Satisfied	Could have skipped those last few bites.
4. Slightly satisfied	I feel satisfied with not one bit of fullness.
5. Neutral	I'm not hungry or full.
6. Slightly hungry	I guess I'm about ready to eat, or I could have a few more bites.
7. Hungry	I'm really ready for another meal.
8. Very hungry	I'm definitely ready for a big meal!
9. Extremely hungry	I can't do one more thing until I eat.
10. Famished (ready to pass out)	Don't talk to me until I eat—I could eat my shirt!

THE DIY PLAN

In the DIY plan, I've controlled the calories and portions for you—that's why the plan says things like "1 cup blueberries," not "all the blueberries you can eat." Portions keep calories under control. What I am giving you in this diet is an outline to get the most nutrition you possibly can while staying within some calorie parameters.

So all you have to do is focus on the most nutritious foods and follow my guidelines. Choose foods from the building blocks (and the proper portions) designated for each meal by using the food charts in this chapter, always following the portion guide. Since I've done the weighing and measuring, you just have to choose foods and add up your ORAC points. No counting calories!

And if the food you want to eat—let's say your favorite breakfast cereal—isn't listed, just pay close attention to the portion sizes associated with similiar items. (This is especially critical for both starches and fats, since both are so easily overeaten. How fast can you down a giant bag of pretzels for 400 calories? Or tear away at an over-500-calorie bagel with 200 calories' worth of butter on it? Pretty quickly, actually.)

When you select a food, it may not have ORAC points associated with it or may not be listed in this book. For example, you may be traveling and choose to have a bowl of bran flakes (a good choice, by the way), and you notice that there is no ORAC value for it. You can use the "other fiber cereal" as your guideline so that you follow along with your correct portions. But, alas, you don't get any ORAC points for that choice!

Without further ado, if you are the type of person who likes to create your own plan, then this O_2 Do-It-Yourself version of my plan is for you. Start choosing your foods *now!*

The building blocks of the DIY plan include in *total* at breakfast, lunch, and dinner *combined* (as listed below):

- One serving from the starch group
- One serving from the fruit group
- One serving from the milk/yogurt/soy group
- Two "servings" from the veggie group
- Two servings from the lean protein group
- Three servings from the fat group
- Herbs/spices at each meal

Here is how you will allocate your building blocks:

Breakfast
Choose fruit or starch
Choose milk/yogurt/soy
Choose fat or protein
Choose herb/spice

Lunch
Choose vegetable
Choose protein
Choose fat
Choose herb/spice

Dinner
Choose vegetable
Choose protein

Choose fat

Choose herb/spice

Include *snacks* accordingly:

- One O_2 veggie snack from page 91. This includes a vegetable and a fat serving. You can feel free to DIY and choose your own veggies and fat *or* choose from the list that follows.

- One O_2 fruit snack from page 91. This includes a fruit and a fat serving. You can feel free to DIY and choose your own fruit and fat *or* choose from the list that follows.

- *Or* in place of the O_2 fruit snack, you can choose an O_2 power snack from page 92.

Your O_2 Breakthrough:
Should I adjust the O_2 Diet for my weight?

Yes! This plan was created for the person who weighs 150 pounds or less.

If you weigh between 151 and 180 pounds, increase your lean protein serving to 4 to 6 ounces.

If you weigh between 181 and 210 pounds, increase your lean protein serving to 6 to 8 ounces.

If you weigh more than 210 pounds, increase your lean protein serving to 6 to 8 ounces and add one serving of starch to any meal.

Building Your Own O₂ Meals

I have my clients fill out a sample DIY day before leaving my office. Yes, you may feel as if you're in grade school, but as I tell my clients, it's very helpful to give this a practice run. Give it a try!

The Building Blocks	Your Sample DIY Day	ORAC Points
Breakfast Choose fruit or starch Choose milk/yogurt/soy Choose fat or protein *Or* choose an O₂ Phase I breakfast recipe (Chapter 5)		
Snack O₂ veggie snack		
Lunch Choose vegetable Choose protein Choose fat Choose herb/spice *Or* choose an O₂ Phase I lunch recipe (Chapter 5)		
Snack O₂ fruit or power snack		
Dinner Choose vegetable Choose protein Choose fat Choose herb/spice *Or* choose *any* O₂ dinner recipe (Chapter 5)		
TOTAL		

Example O₂ Diet DIY Day

DIY Day 1	ORAC Values
Breakfast	
1 plum	4,100
¾ c fat-free plain yogurt	—
10 almonds	500
½ tsp cinnamon	3,500
Snack	
Green tea	3,000
1 c celery	500
2 tsp almond butter	400
¼ tsp cinnamon	1,750
Lunch	
1 c romaine lettuce, 1 plum tomato, ¼ c carrots, 10 strips yellow bell peppers, ½ c artichoke hearts	500; 300; 225; 500; 7,900
4 oz canned tuna	—
18 pistachios	1,000
1 oz lemon juice, 1 tsp black pepper	400; 600
Snack	
Green tea	3,000
¾ c fat-free plain yogurt	—
1 Tbsp chopped walnuts and ¼ tsp cinnamon	1,900; 1,750
Dinner	
1 c raw spinach, ¼ c red onions (with raspberry vinegar)	500; 400
White meat turkey burger	—
7 walnut halves (on salad)	1,900
½ tsp garlic powder and ½ tsp onion powder (in turkey burger)	100; 50
8 c water with 1 oz lemon juice per cup	3,200
TOTAL	37,975

DIY Day 2	ORAC Values
Breakfast	
1 c blackberries	7,700
1 c soy milk	—
2 Tbsp ground flaxseed	—
1 c ice	—
½ tsp cinnamon	3,500
Snack	
1 c green tea	3,000
1 c red bell peppers	1,200
8 pecans	2,500
Lunch	
1 c raw spinach, 1 c red onions, and 1 c cucumbers	500; 800; 200
4 oz grilled chicken	—
2 tsp olive oil and fig vinegar (on salad)	100
1 tsp dried oregano (on chicken)	3,600
Snack	
1 c green tea	3,000
¾ c edamame	5,400
¼ tsp black pepper and sea salt, to taste (on edamame)	150
Dinner	
1 c steamed broccoli	3,800
1 oz lemon juice and sea salt	400
1 whole tomato and ¼ avocado (salad)	300; 700
4 oz grilled scallops	—
½ tsp cumin (on scallops)	800
8 c water with 1 oz lemon juice per cup	3,200
TOTAL	40,550

(continued)

Example O₂ Diet DIY Day—*cont.*

DIY Day 3	ORAC Values
Breakfast	
½ c oatmeal	600
1 c skim milk	—
8 pecan halves	2,500
½ tsp cinnamon	3,500
Snack	
1 c green tea	3,000
Veggie Crunch (page 91)	2,600
Lunch	
1 c steamed green beans	800
4 oz grilled salmon	—
10 chopped almonds (on green beans)	500
2 sprigs dill (on salmon)	44
Snack	
1 c green tea	3,000
¾ c fat-free plain yogurt with ½ c canned pumpkin puree, sprinkled with ½ teaspoon cinnamon	3,800
Dinner	
1 c broiled asparagus	3,000
1 c chopped romaine lettuce	500
½ c beets	—
½ c carrots	450
½ c celery	250
¼ c cucumber	50
Water chestnuts	—
4 oz roasted chicken (no skin)	—
2 tsp olive oil and balsamic vinegar (on salad)	100
1 tsp rosemary (on chicken)	364
8 c water with 1 oz lemon juice per cup	3,200
TOTAL	31,758

DIY Day 4	ORAC Values
Breakfast	
1 slice pumpernickel bread	500
Stonyfield Farm Light Smoothie	—
Omega-3-enriched scrambled eggs (1 yolk, 3 whites)	—
½ tsp paprika (on eggs)	200
Snack	
1 cup green tea	3,000
Carrots and 2 tsp peanut butter with ¼ tsp cinnamon	3,000
Lunch	
1 c crudités of red and yellow peppers, carrots, zucchini	500 (average of the vegetables)
1 c lentil soup	15,000
3 Tbsp guacamole	—
½ tsp cumin (in soup)	800
Snack	
1 cup green tea	3,000
Green apple	7,100
2 tsp peanut butter	400
Dinner	
1 bunch sautéed broccoli rabe	6,800
1 c red leaf lettuce	700
½ c carrots	200
¼ c mushrooms	—
¼ c red onions	400
Pork tenderloin	—
2 tsp olive oil (for broccoli rabe)	100
1 tsp thyme (on pork)	200
1 oz lemon juice, 1 tsp black pepper, and kosher salt, to taste (on salad)	400
8 c water with 1 oz lemon juice per cup	3,200
TOTAL	44,780

Keep in mind as you use the charts below that the US Agricultural Research Service performed its tests on 100 grams of each food. I have taken these numbers and converted them to ounces and then converted to the proper portions for this plan. The numbers have been rounded for your convenience.

FRUIT

By now, I've convinced you that fruit is an amazing source of antioxidants. (I bet I had you at blueberries, didn't I?) But that's not the only reason I'm asking you to eat it. Fresh fruits are also high in fiber, which fills you up. The high water content of whole fruit helps, too, so that a fruit snack can keep you feeling satisfied for a long time! *Fresh* fruit is always my first choice. Substituting fruit juice not only deprives you of fiber but also makes it all too easy to overconsume calories. Dried fruit, too, is higher in calories than fresh fruit and often has added sugar (always opt for "no sugar added") and sulfur (a preservative). The exceptions? Some high-antioxidant fruits, such as cranberries, currants, and goji berries, are easier to find in dried form. Others, such as acai and pomegranate, are easier to find as juices. In those cases, pay extra attention to the portion sizes—there is no need to eat any additional fruit beyond what I've suggested, and eating more may slow down your weight loss.

Fruit	Serving	ORAC Value
Blueberries	1 c	9,700
Cranberries (raw)	1 c	9,600
Red Delicious apple	1	7,800
Blackberries	1 c	7,700
Granny Smith apple	1	7,100
Raspberries	1 c	6,000
Strawberries	1 c	5,400
Gala apple	1	5,200
Pear	1	5,200
Fuji apple	1	4,700
Plum	1	4,100
Cherries	¾ c	3,500
Guava, red-fleshed	1 c	3,300
Orange	1	3,000
Figs	2	2,700
Peach	1	2,700
Applesauce	½ c	2,400

Fruit	Serving	ORAC Value
Guava, white-fleshed	½ c	2,100
Grapefruit, pink or red	½	1,900
Pineapple, extra sweet variety	1 c	1,500
Tangerine	1	1,400
Apricot	3	1,200
Peach, dried (no sugar added)	¼ c	1,200
Red grapes	1 c	1,200
Nectarine	1	1,100
Banana	1	1,000
White or green grapes	1 c	1,000
Pineapple	1 c	900
Mango	½ c	800
Kiwi	1	700
Papaya	1 c	500
Cantaloupe	1 c	500
Honeydew	1 c	400
Watermelon	1 c	200

Dried Fruit	Serving	ORAC Value
Cranberries, dried	2 Tbsp	2,100
Prunes	3	1,900
Currants	2 Tbsp	1,100
Raisins	2 Tbsp	600

STARCHES

The following starches not only give us a little antioxidant punch but also provide fiber, B vitamins, and a little protein—and for many people, they're the most satisfying part of a meal. Unfortunately, some starchy foods don't make it onto the ORAC scale. This does not mean they are not "good" foods. In fact, some of them are my favorites. That's why I list quinoa, whole wheat pasta, brown and wild rice, kamut, and millet here—you may not be able to add in ORAC points, but I promise you will be getting a whole lot of nutrients. Just pack in your ORAC points elsewhere. And if you end up with a piece of white bread (ah, dare I say that!) at your favorite brasserie, use the "other breads" portion to keep the calories in check, even if you don't get to add ORAC points.

Starch	Serving	ORAC Value
Cereal		
Oat bran flakes	¾ c	800
Popcorn, air-popped	5 c	700
Instant oatmeal	1 packet	600
Wheat germ	3 Tbsp	—
Other high-fiber cereal	½–¾ c	—
Bread/Crackers		
Pumpernickel bread	1 slice	500
Oat nut bread	1 slice	400
Whole grain/seven-grain bread	1 slice	400
Other breads	1 slice	—
High-fiber crackers	3–5 crackers	—
Starchy Vegetable		
Sweet potato with skin	1 medium	2,400
Red potato with skin	1 small	1,800
White potato with skin	½ medium	1,600
Russet potato with skin	½ medium	1,500
Corn	¾ c	700
Butternut squash	1 c	600
Pumpkin	1 c	600
Peas	¾ c	400
Legume		
Black beans	½ c	7,800
Kidney beans	½ c	7,800
Lentils	½ c	7,500
Pinto beans	½ c	7,000
Black-eyed peas	½ c	3,600
Chickpeas	½ c	800
Split peas	½ c	500
Other legumes	½ c	—
Other		
Brown rice	⅓ c	—
Bulgur	⅓ c	—
Kamut	⅓ c	—
Millet	⅓ c	—
Quinoa	⅓ c	—
Whole wheat pasta	⅓ c	—
Wild rice	⅓ c	—

MILK, YOGURT, AND OTHER

Wait, you're probably thinking—*where are my ORAC points?* Milk and yogurt are not filled with the traditional nutrients that give foods an ORAC value. But they still play a crucial role in your diet. The following options are highest in calcium and protein with as little sugar as possible. Even though chocolate milk is a bit high in sugar, I have put it on the list because the added ORAC points are too valuable to pass up. Plus I find that many people who turn up their noses at a glass of milk will happily suck down chocolate milk. And for you gym rats out there, chocolate milk is an excellent recovery drink! Note that I do *not* include chocolate milk in your 2-week plan, because I want to keep your sugar intake low. So if you are doing the DIY, for the first 2 weeks, avoid it. However, as you continue on the O_2 Diet for life, chocolate milk may be a nice option for an O_2 power snack.

Milk/Yogurt/Other	Serving	ORAC Value
Low-fat (1 percent) chocolate milk	½ c	1,600
Fat-free Greek yogurt (plain)	¾ c	—
Low-fat (1 percent) or fat-free cottage cheese	½ c	—
Soy milk (plain)	1 c	—
Skim milk	1 c	0
Other milk (almond, rice, hemp)	1 c	0

Your O_2 Breakthrough:
How many points for a salad?

Calculating the ORAC points of a mixed salad can seem daunting—and frankly, if you tried to break down every salad into all its measurable components, you might go completely insane. I use this rule of thumb: One cup of mixed salad (the amount you'd be served as a side salad at most restaurants) is likely to contain mostly lettuces, relatively low in ORAC points, and very small amounts of other vegetables—maybe some red cabbage, carrot bits, cucumber, tomatoes, and a radish or two. I calculate those salads at 850 ORAC points, on average. For an entrée-size salad, I'd use 2 cups (1,700 ORAC points) and juice up the ORAC value by adding things like red kidney beans, artichoke hearts, and nuts—all of which are listed in this chapter's charts. Don't forget you can download the ORAC points chart at www.theO2diet.com and carry it with you and/or use the O_2 ORAC calculator online at www.theO2diet.com .

VEGETABLES

Veggies are of course high in antioxidants, but they also contain fiber and even a little protein. Remember, though, you do want to eat a variety. Mix it up and learn to love your veggies—all veggies! I also want to point out that some very nutritious vegetables—even some of my faves—have not been tested by the ARS for ORAC value. Other amazing greens I suggest are dandelion greens, Swiss chard, and bok choy. Be creative: Throw some mushrooms into your next salad or on your next turkey burger. Water chestnuts and jicama add crunch that can't be beat in a salad.

Vegetable	Serving (At least! Go for 1 serving as a snack and 2 to 3 times this serving amount at a meal.)	ORAC Value
Artichoke hearts	½ c	7,900
Broccoli rabe	1 bunch	6,800
Red cabbage (cooked)	½ c	2,400
Radish (raw)	1 c	2,000
Broccoli (cooked)	½ c	1,900
Kale (raw)	1 c	1,770
Onion (raw)	1 c	1,600
Red cabbage (raw)	1 c	1,600
Asparagus (cooked)	½ c	1,500
Green bell peppers (raw)	1 c	1,400
Salsa	½ c	1,300
Spinach (cooked)	½ c	1,300
Broccoli (raw)	1 c	1,200
Red bell peppers (raw)	1 c	1,200
Brussels sprouts (cooked)	½ c	980
Carrots (raw)	1 c	900
Tomato sauce	½ c	900
Beet greens (shredded)	1 c	800
Boston/Bibb lettuce (shredded)	1 c	800
Cauliflower (raw)	1 c	800
Eggplant (raw)	1 c	800
Green beans (raw)	1 c	800
Red onions	½ c	800
Alfalfa sprouts	1 c	700

(continued)

The O₂ Diet

Vegetable	Serving (At least! Go for 1 serving as a snack and 2 to 3 times this serving amount at a meal.)	ORAC Value
Red leaf lettuce (shredded)	1 c	700
Vegetable juice	4 oz	700
Cabbage (cooked)	1/2 c	600
Tomato juice	1/2 c	600
Yellow onions (cooked)	1/2 c	550
Celery	1 c	500
Green leaf lettuce (shredded)	1 c	500
Onion, sweet	1/4	500
Red tomatoes (cooked)	1/2 cup	500
Romaine lettuce (shredded)	1 c	500
Spinach (raw)	1 c	500
Yellow bell peppers (raw)	10 strips	500
Cauliflower (cooked)	1/2 c	400
Leeks (raw)	1 c	400
Plum tomato (raw)	1	300
Iceberg lettuce (shredded)	1 c	300
Carrots (cooked)	1/2 c	200
Cucumber with peel (sliced)	1 c	200
Eggplant (cooked)	1/2 c	200
Fennel, bulb (raw)	1 c	200
Zucchini (raw)	1 c	100
Other veggies	1/2 c cooked or 1 c raw	—

LEAN PROTEINS

Protein is satisfying. The protein sources listed in the table on page 84 are the leanest. If you find yourself hungry at a meal and have already eaten your portion, feel free to have an extra ounce. Just make sure you're listening to your HQ and *stop* when you feel "slightly satisfied."

But when it comes to cheese, hold up! I do list some cheese options, and cheese appears in a few of the recipes that follow. Cheese is delicious, full of calcium, and a good protein source, but it's also a leading source of saturated fat in our diets (that's not good). And because cheeses are so calorie dense, they can wreak real caloric damage. When you choose cheese, avoid full-fat varieties, and pay close attention to the portions I recommend (see Your O₂ Breakthrough on page 72 for more information).

Lean Protein	Serving	ORAC Value
Poultry		
Chicken breast	3–4 oz	—
Cornish hen	3–4 oz	—
Turkey breast	3–4 oz	—
Turkey bacon	3–4 oz	—
Turkey burger	3–4 oz	—
Turkey jerky	3–4 oz	—
Chicken/turkey meatballs	3–4 oz	—
Chicken hot dog	3–4 oz	—
Chicken sausage	3–4 oz	—
Turkey hot dog	3–4 oz	—
Seafood		
Cod	3–4 oz	—
Flounder	3–4 oz	—
Clams	3–4 oz	—
Halibut	3–4 oz	—
King crab	3–4 oz	—
Lobster	3–4 oz	—
Mahimahi	3–4 oz	—
Mussels	3–4 oz	—
Red snapper	3–4 oz	—
Salmon (wild)	3–4 oz	—
Scallops	3–4 oz	—
Shrimp	3–4 oz	—
Sardines	3–4 oz	—
Sole	3–4 oz	—
Swordfish	3–4 oz	—
Trout	3–4 oz	—
Tuna	3–4 oz	—
Tuna (canned chunk light in water)	3–4 oz	—
Tuna (canned chunk light in olive oil)	3–4 oz	—
Tuna	3–4 oz	—
Tuna jerky	3–4 oz	—
Salmon jerky	3–4 oz	—

(continued)

Lean Protein	Serving	ORAC Value
Meat		
Ground beef, 95% lean	3–4 oz	—
Beef tenderloin	3–4 oz	—
Lamb loin	3–4 oz	—
Roast beef (deli slices)	3–4 oz	—
Game		
Ostrich	3–4 oz	—
Venison	3–4 oz	—
Bison	3–4 oz	—
Pork		
Ham, extra lean	3–4 oz	—
Pork, center loin chop	3–4 oz	—
Pork cutlet	3–4 oz	—
Pork tenderloin	3–4 oz	—
Vegetarian Options		
Black beans (or black bean soup)	1 c	15,600
Kidney beans	1 c	15,600
Pinto beans	1 c	15,000
Lentils	1 c	14,000
Black-eyed peas	1 c	7,300
Edamame (soybeans)	¾ c	5,400
Chickpeas	1 c	1,700
Split peas	1 c	1,000
Hummus	4 Tbsp	400
Egg whites (Egg Beaters)	4–6 egg whites	—
Firm tofu	4 oz	—
Tempeh	4 oz	—
Veggie burger	1 patty	—
Cottage cheese (low fat or fat free)	¾ c	—
Reduced-fat feta cheese	2 oz	—
Part-skim fresh mozzarella cheese	2 oz	—
Parmesan cheese	3 Tbsp	—

FATS

With all the talk about people being overweight, it's easy to forget that fat isn't just good for us, it's essential! We need about one-third of our calories to come from it every day. But fat provides more than double the calories per gram than protein and carbohydrates, so portion control with regards to fat is crucial to monitor. My focus is on eating the most nutritious fats—including monounsaturated and polyunsaturated fats and essential fatty acids such as the omega-3s.

Fat	Serving	ORAC Value
Pecans	8 halves	2,500
Walnuts	7 halves	1,900
Hazelnuts	8	1,000
Pistachios	18	1,000
Avocado	¼	700
Guacamole	2 Tbsp	700
Almonds	10	500
Almond butter	2 tsp	500
Peanuts	15	500
Peanut butter	2 tsp	500
Cashews	8	200
Olive oil, extra virgin	2 tsp	100
Brazil nuts	2	100
Pine nuts	1 Tbsp	100
Macadamia nuts	3	100
Oil-based salad dressing	1 Tbsp	—
Other oils (walnut, grapeseed, canola, sunflower, flax)	2 tsp	—
Flaxseed	2 Tbsp	—
Pumpkin seeds	1 Tbsp	—
Coconut (shredded)	¼ c	—
Cottage cheese (low fat or fat free)	¼ c	—
Reduced-fat feta cheese	1 oz	—
Part-skim fresh mozzarella cheese	1 oz	—
Parmesan cheese	1 Tbsp	—
One whole egg	—	—

BEVERAGES

Drink up! As I have already discussed, being properly hydrated is key to being energetic and functioning at your best as well as helping aid in weight loss. The alcoholic beverages listed below are considered *conscious indulgences* that you will incorporate in Phase III. Substitute the juices for a fruit serving. The "free" beverages—well, those you can chug!

Beverage	Serving	ORAC Value
Wine (Incorporate alcohol as a *conscious indulgence*.)		
Sangria (See recipe on page 98.)	4 oz	11,900
Cabernet	5 oz	7,400
Red	5 oz	5,700
Rosé	5 oz	1,500
White	5 oz	600
Tea (Drink up—no calories here!)		
Green tea	1 c	3,000
Black tea	1 c	2,700
Other herbal teas	1 c	—
Juice (to be consumed in lieu of whole fruit)		
Blueberry juice	½ c	3,600
Pomegranate juice	½ c	2,900
Concord grape juice	½ c	2,900
Prune juice	½ c	2,600
Red grape juice	½ c	2,300
Cranberry–Concord grape juice	½ c	1,800
White grapefruit juice	½ c	1,500
Cranberry juice	½ c	1,100
White grape juice	½ c	1,000
Orange juice	½ c	900
Pineapple juice	½ c	700
Apple juice	½ c	500
White cranberry juice	½ c	300
"Free" Beverage (Calories minimal—add freely to water, seltzer, or tea.)		
Lemon juice	1 oz	400
Lime juice	1 oz	300

"Free" Beverages with an O_2 Punch!

These ORAC values are based on my favorite beverages (see Your O_2 Shopping List on page 167). ORAC values will vary depending on how you prepare them, but they're "free," so have fun!

Iced Green Tea

Steep 2 green tea bags in 8 ounces boiling water 1 to 3 minutes with 2 lemon slices. Add 4 ounces cold water and ice cubes and 2 mint leaves.

ORAC Value: 6,000

Cucumber Water with Ginger

Combine 10 ounces water with 3 or 4 $\frac{1}{4}$-inch slices seedless cucumber with skin and let stand 10 minutes. Add pinch of dry ginger or fresh ginger.

ORAC Value: 100

Blueberry Iced Tea

Steep 2 blueberry tea bags in 8 ounces boiling water 1 to 3 minutes with 2 lime slices. Add 4 ounces cold water and ice cubes.

ORAC Value: 1,000

Sparkling Raspberry "Soda"

Steep 2 raspberry tea bags in 8 ounces boiling water 1 to 3 minutes. Add 6 ounces club soda and ice.

ORAC Value: 1,000

Iced Coffee

Mix $\frac{1}{8}$ teaspoon ground nutmeg and $\frac{1}{8}$ teaspoon ground cinnamon into 8 ounces of brewed hot coffee. Then, pour over ice and add $\frac{1}{2}$ teaspoon vanilla extract.

ORAC Value: 875

HERBS AND SPICES

Spices are an incredibly rich source of antioxidants—a teaspoon of cinnamon has more antioxidant value as a half cup of blueberries, and turmeric is on par with raspberries. The phenols and other antioxidant properties are linked to all kinds of health perks, including cinnamon's ability to help stabilize blood sugar; oregano's antimicrobial effect, which may prevent ulcers; and turmeric's ability to reduce inflammation and maybe even ward off cancer. Besides preparing food recipes that call for allspice, cinnamon, cloves, ginger, marjoram, mint, oregano, rosemary, and sage, think of ways to use herbs and spices in beverages: Sprinkling ½ teaspoon of cinnamon on your coffee grounds before brewing will add 3,500 ORAC points, while mixing ½ teaspoon of dried ginger in your lemon water will add 250 ORAC points.

Discard spices that are more than 2 years old, and store spices in a dark cupboard—being too near the stove or sunlight will zap their power. (Not sure how old it is? If it's a McCormick spice, go to www.mccormick.com, click on Spices 101, and you can type in the product code to find out when it was bottled.)

Herb/Spice	Serving	ORAC Value
Cinnamon, ground	1 tsp	7,000
Cloves, ground	1 tsp	6,600
Oregano, dried	1 tsp	3,600
Turmeric, ground	1 tsp	3,500
Cumin seed	1 tsp	1,600
Curry powder	1 tsp	1,000
Mustard seed, yellow	1 tsp	1,000
Chili powder	1 tsp	600
Pepper, black	1 tsp	600
Basil, dried	1 tsp	500
Ginger, ground	1 tsp	500
Sage, fresh	2 tsp	500
Oregano, fresh	2 tsp	400
Paprika	1 tsp	400
Parsley, dried	1 tsp	400
Peppermint, fresh	2 Tbsp	400
Rosemary, dried	1 tsp	400

(continued)

Herb/Spice	Serving	ORAC Value
Tarragon, fresh	2 tsp	310
Gingerroot, raw	1 tsp	300
Coriander (cilantro) leaves, raw	¼ c	200
Garlic powder or raw	1 tsp	200
Thyme, fresh	1 tsp	200
Basil, fresh (chopped)	1 Tbsp	100
Cardamom	1 tsp	100
Onion powder	1 tsp	100
Parsley, raw	1 Tbsp	100
Dill weed, fresh	5 sprigs	100
Chives, raw (chopped)	1 tsp	100
Poppy seed	1 tsp	100

CONDIMENTS

Condiments are an easy way to flavor up your favorite foods. However, the calories can add up quick! For instance, ketchup, although it has an ORAC value of 100 per tablespoon, does have 15 calories for that same spoonful. So make sure to stick to the serving size and don't think you can have a little burger with your ketchup—instead, have a little ketchup with your burger. Feel free to pour on low-cal and no-cal condiments like vinegars. In the shopping list in Chapter 8, you will see more condiments that I suggest to use on your food as "free" flavor.

Condiment	Serving	ORAC Value
Salsa	½ c	1,300
Apple vinegar	1 Tbsp	100
Ketchup	1 Tbsp	100
Red wine vinegar	1 Tbsp	100

SNACKS

As discussed earlier, snacks are an integral part of the O$_2$ Diet. They help keep you feeling satisfied and make sure your metabolism stays revved.

I want you to choose:

- An O$_2$ veggie snack *and* an O$_2$ fruit snack

or

- An O$_2$ veggie snack *and* an O$_2$ power snack

O$_2$ Veggie Snacks (or Choose Your Own Veggie and Fat)

ORAC GOAL: OVER 2,000

Celery, 2 teaspoons almond butter, and ¼ teaspoon cinnamon: 2,700

Sliced red bell peppers and 8 pecan halves: 3,100

Artichoke, 2 teaspoons olive oil, and 2 tablespoons lemon juice: 8,600

Carrots, 2 teaspoons peanut butter, and ¼ teaspoon cinnamon: 3,000

Yellow and red bell peppers, ¼ avocado with 1 tablespoon lime juice, and 1 teaspoon chopped cilantro for a quick guacamole: 2,000

Veggie Crunch: Chopped carrots, sliced radish, red and yellow bell peppers, and chopped cucumber mixed with 2 teaspoons walnut oil and fig vinegar to taste: 2,600

Blanched asparagus dipped in ¼ cup jarred salsa mixed with 2 tablespoons chopped avocado or 2 teaspoons chopped cashews: 2,200

Cucumber Boat: 1 Kirby cucumber, halved and scooped, filled with ⅓ cup halved grape tomatoes and 1 tablespoon chopped red onion and tossed with 2 teaspoons extra virgin olive oil and red wine vinegar to taste: 2,100

O$_2$ Fruit Snacks (or Choose Your Own Fruit and Fat)

ORAC GOAL: OVER 3,000

Green apple, 2 teaspoons peanut butter, and ¼ teaspoon cinnamon: 9,200

Sliced pear, 1 tablespoon chopped walnuts, and ¼ teaspoon cinnamon: 7,900

Plum and 2 teaspoons almond butter: 4,700

1 cup blueberries and 8 pecan halves: 12,200

1 cup blackberries and 18 pistachios: 8,700

¾ cup cherries and 10 almonds: 4,000

2 figs and 8 hazelnuts: 3,700

2 tablespoons dried cranberries and 8 pecan halves: 3,600

2 tablespoons currants and 8 pecan halves: 3,600

O₂ Power Snacks
(or Choose Your Own Yogurt and Fruit or Yogurt and Fat)

ORAC GOAL: OVER 1,000

½ cup reduced-fat chocolate milk with 1 cup raspberries: 7,600

1 cup green tea with 6 ounces steamed soy milk and ¼ teaspoon cinnamon: 4,700

6 ounces fat-free plain yogurt and ½ cup canned pumpkin puree sprinkled with ½ teaspoon cinnamon: 3,800

4 ounces fat-free plain yogurt with ½ ounce dark chocolate and ¼ cup raspberries: 5,000

6 ounces fat-free plain yogurt with 8 walnut halves and ¼ teaspoon cinnamon: 4,000

6 ounces fat-free plain yogurt with 2 ounces pomegranate juice and ½ cup blueberries: 6,300

1 cup edamame with ¼ teaspoon black pepper and sea salt to taste: 10,900

6 ounces fat-free plain yogurt with 2 teaspoons peanut butter and ¼ teaspoon cinnamon: 2,200

½ cup fat-free cottage cheese with ½ cup cantaloupe, ½ cup blackberries, and 1 teaspoon finely chopped mint: 4,100

1 peach cut in half and spread with 1 ounce fat-free ricotta cheese and ¼ teaspoon cinnamon: 4,500

Your O₂ Breakthrough:
Six-course tasting menu got you down?

Got a fried-food hangover? Should you skip breakfast? Eat 4 quarts of blueberries? Here's the answer: You should get right back to your O₂ life. As I say, every meal is a Monday morning—an opportunity to eat well. Take each meal individually. You made a mistake; now *move on!* You can up your ORAC intake by indulging in some "free" O₂ power snacks. The snacks' ORAC levels are not too high, but the calories are nada! Next, have an "O₂ shot." Instead of those few pieces of gum you may chew at your desk, go for a shot of ORAC to help put you back in the zone. If your ORAC intake was low one day, use the "free" O₂ power snacks to up your score the next—and of course aim for the highest ORAC foods to balance you as well.

5 cups air-popped popcorn sprinkled with ½ teaspoon chili powder and sea salt to taste: 1,000

¼ cup black bean dip and celery sticks: 4,400

6 ounces fat-free plain yogurt with ½ cup unsweetened applesauce: 2,400

¼ cup fat-free plain yogurt with ¼ avocado and ¼ teaspoon cumin, served with ½ cup radishes: 2,100

2 part-skim mozzarella cheese sticks dipped in ¼ cup marinara sauce seasoned with ¼ teaspoon oregano: 1,300

Beet and carrot chips: 1 medium beet, sliced; 1 tablespoon extravirgin olive oil; 1 cup carrot slices; 1 teaspoon cinnamon. Place veggies on a baking sheet, brush with olive oil, and sprinkle with cinnamon. Bake 8 to 12 minutes at 350°F, or to desired crispness: 9,400

1 cup strawberries drizzled with 1 tablespoon dark chocolate chunks melted in the microwave: 8,400

"Free" O₂ Power Snacks

A little low on your ORAC points today? It's okay! You can power up with a few free snacks and drinks without upping your calories.

Cabbage Slaw

½ cup red cabbage

½ cup white cabbage

2 teaspoons Dijon mustard

1 tablespoon apple cider vinegar

Combine ingredients.

ORAC Value: 2,200

Cucumber Salad

1 or 2 sliced seedless cucumbers with skin

Fig vinegar

Place cucumbers in small bowl, cover with fig vinegar, and let marinate for 1 hour. Drain vinegar.

ORAC Value: 400

O₂ Shots

How many times have you grabbed a butterscotch candy from the bowl at the nail salon? The O₂ shots below will provide no more calories than that little candy, yet they'll supply a nice ORAC punch. So forget the wasted calories—give your teeth a rest and power up!

6 ounces club soda with 2 ounces cranberry juice: 600

8 ounces water with 1 ounce lemon and 1 ounce acai juice: 4,200

8 ounces water with 2 fresh mint leaves and 1 ounce pomegranate juice: 2,700

O₂ phase III: weeks 3 and 4

At this point, you should be in full ORAC swing! Eating 30,000 points per day is not nearly as difficult as you had thought it would be. And now you get to add one ORAC starch or fruit serving per day. Be sure to pay special attention to the ORAC starches, such as sweet potato, and the nutrient-rich starches, such as quinoa. You can also choose any O₂ breakfast, lunch, or dinner from Chapter 5. Finally, indulge! Choose one *conscious indulgence* per week (consume no other alcohol unless it is your *conscious indulgence*).

O₂ PHASE III GUIDELINES

In Phase III, you can choose DIY options or repeat the first 2 weeks from Phase II. The guidelines are the same as for Phase II, but with a few more perks! Here are the basics again, in case you need a reminder.

- Eat 30,000 (or more) ORAC points per day (within the diet guidelines).

- Begin each day with a glass of water with lemon

- Have at least 8 glasses of water per day and aim to add 1 ounce of lemon juice to each glass.

- Drink at least 2 cups of green tea per day.

- Use herbs and spices as much as possible. Aim to add them to breakfast, lunch, and dinner daily.

Your O$_2$ Breakthrough:
Carbs, fats, and protein

By now you're probably wondering . . . is the O$_2$ Diet high carb? Low fat? High protein? None of the above! The O$_2$ Diet is perfectly proportioned to give you the proper ratio of carbs to fat to protein while paying careful attention to anti-oxidants, other nutrients, and calories. If you follow the basic building blocks of each meal and stick to the portions I've outlined, you will end up with a diet that is almost equal parts carbs, fat, and protein (with carbs having a bit of an edge).

Protein provides the body with power in many ways. It is the structural component of all cells of the body. Protein can function as an enzyme, a hormone, and a transporter/carrier. Protein also provides satiety, meaning that it helps to keep us feeling full. The protein foods I recommend are mostly lean protein sources. You can get the same amount of protein from a lean piece of meat as you will from a fatty one—and we certainly do not need the extra artery-clogging calories from fatty cuts of meat.

Carbs provide energy to all cells of our bodies, particularly our brains! What good are all those brain-boosting antioxidants if you don't have energy to use them? But remember, you get carbs from starches, fruit, yogurt, and even vegetables. In the O$_2$ plan, you eat just the right amount of carbs from sources that provide you with other important nutrients. This is why the majority of your carbs will come from fruit, yogurt, and veggies. The carbohydrates you get from starch will be the highest ORAC starches and/or the highest fiber choices.

So where does fat fit in? You need fat! Our bodies need some fat to function properly. Fat deficiency causes our skin to be dry, makes our hair brittle, often leaves us constipated (need I say more about how that makes us feel?), and can cause gastrointestinal distress, menstrual abnormalities, fatigue, anemia, headaches, and even memory loss. Fat helps us absorb certain vitamins and minerals (some of them antioxidants) properly. We also need fat to burn fat! Finally, fat makes food taste palatable, which is what gives us a feeling of greater satisfaction with a meal or snack. The problem, though, is that that's the same quality that makes us want to overeat fat! That's why we need to pay close attention to eating the right fats—healthy fats from mono- and polyunsaturated sources and omega-3s—and the right portion of fats. A little fat goes a long way toward helping us feel satisfied and enjoy our food. This is why you will consume a small portion of fat throughout the day on the plan.

- Use your O$_2$ Life Journal to help you track your food and ORAC points (see page 204 or visit www.theO2diet.com to download the journal and an ORAC points guide).

- Continue to aim for those 7 to 8 hours of sleep per night. Make a nap date if you fall short.

- Whatever type of exerciser you may be, be consistent. Put your workouts in your calendar like doctor appointments, and stick to them.

- Pamper yourself as you did during the cleanse. Hopefully, cleansing and moisturizing your skin have become habits.

And then in Phase III, you can add:

- One starch or fruit. (For example, a sweet potato with dinner. Yum!)

- One O$_2$ *conscious indulgence.*

Are you the kind of person who skips right over the word *indulgence*, thinking the "tougher" you are on yourself, the quicker you'll lose weight? Over the years, my work with clients has proven that indulgences are very important—without them, people build up a gradual sense of deprivation that usually culminates in a major binge. (The names Ben and Jerry come up regularly!) Treat yourself right on the O$_2$ Diet. You'll be surprised to learn that even decadent foods have an ORAC value. The key is to use them wisely, since the calories add up fast. Here's a list of sweet treats with ORAC values and the correct portion of an *indulgence.*

Indulgence	Serving	ORAC Value
Baking chocolate, unsweetened, squares	1 square	14,500
Dark chocolate	1 oz	5,900
Semisweet chocolate	1 oz	5,100
Chocolate syrup	2 Tbsp	2,500
Milk chocolate	1 oz	2,200
Cocoa powder	1 Tbsp	100

O$_2$ CONSCIOUS INDULGENCES

A *conscious indulgence* is a controlled indulgence. Here are some of my favorite combos. If you choose a non-ORAC conscious indulgence, try to keep it to three bites or 100 to 150 calories.

Hot chocolate: 1 cup reduced-fat chocolate milk heated with 2 mint leaves: 3,300

Chocolate pear: 1 sliced pear dipped in ½ ounce melted dark chocolate with a pinch of ground cloves: 8,900

Chocolate-covered figs: 2 figs dipped in ½ ounce melted dark chocolate, then allowed to cool and harden: 5,700

"Banana split": ½ banana, sliced lengthwise, topped with a mixture of 2 tablespoons fat-free plain yogurt, 1 teaspoon agave syrup, and 8 chopped pecans: 5,100

Coconut pudding: ¼ cup fat-free cottage cheese with 1 tablespoon light coconut milk, 1 tablespoon shredded coconut, and 1 chopped date: 1,500

Chocolate-covered pecans: 8 pecans dipped in ½ ounce melted dark chocolate, then allowed to cool and harden: 8,100

Warm pineapple: 1 cup extrasweet pineapple chunks or thinly sliced pineapple rounds broiled (or grilled) about 5 minutes in a baking dish positioned 4 inches from the heat; turn the slices once. Serve tossed with 8 chopped hazelnuts: 2,600

Coconut sundae: ½ cup fat-free plain yogurt with ½ ounce melted dark chocolate and 1 tablespoon coconut shavings: 3,000

You can also choose to indulge in an alcoholic beverage. See the ORAC values for wine and sangria listed in the "Beverages" section. If you are not a fan of wine and prefer another cocktail, feel free to indulge, but be aware that most alcoholic drinks offer no ORAC points. As a rule of thumb, stay away from the high-sugar drinks and stick with a glass of wine, a wine spritzer, a light beer, or a vodka and soda. My fave? Club soda with a splash of vodka and a whole lot of squeezed lime for a nice O$_2$ kick! Also check out the delicious high-ORAC Blackberry-Thyme Margarita recipe on page 146. And my personal recipe for an O$_2$ indulgence . . .

Sangria

1 bottle Cabernet

$1\frac{1}{2}$ tablespoons agave syrup

1 orange, sliced

1 lemon, sliced

1 medium peach, sliced

1 medium-firm pear, sliced

1 cup club soda

Mix all ingredients together. If you are in the mood to have a little more fun, you can up the ORAC value of this cocktail by adding chunks of pineapple, raspberries, or slices of green apple.

ORAC Value: 11,900

THE O$_2$ DIET DINING-OUT GUIDELINES

Dining out intimidates most dieters. Some of my clients told me that they avoid restaurants altogether when they're trying to "be good." Others go from feast to famine, and all of their healthy habits go out the window. But there are very simple guidelines you can follow to make sure that dining out doesn't mean sipping hot water while everyone else enjoys a hearty meal; nor does it mean eating the entire bread basket, four appetizers and dessert. Dining out the O$_2$ way can be easy if you follow these few simple guidelines.

Before you eat

- Never go to a restaurant when your HQ is close to 10 (starving). You have already slowed your metabolism, and chances are you will make poor choices for your main course (as well as eat the entire bread basket). Have a small snack beforehand, so you walk into the restaurant with your HQ around 6, tops.

- Never skip meals knowing you are going out for a nice dinner or to your favorite restaurant. This almost guarantees that you'll overeat and slow your metabolism!

- Always drink a large glass of water before you get to the restaurant or as soon as you arrive. This will fill you up slightly and make you feel healthy.

At the restaurant

- Look for high-ORAC, high-fiber starch options, such as whole wheat bread or sweet potato.

- Choose leaner sources of protein or high-omega-3 sources such as scallops or salmon. Stay away from things fried and sautéed. Order foods that are baked, boiled, steamed, poached, roasted, or grilled. But be careful! Believe it or not, foods that are poached may be poached in fat! The same goes for boiled foods. Don't be afraid to ask what the food is poached or boiled in.

- Substitute heart-healthy high-ORAC fats such as olive oil and walnut oil for saturated fats like butter.

- Order dressings and sauces on the side and *you* control the portions.

- Fill up on the highest-ORAC veggies available. Instead of diving into the bread basket, ask for an order of steamed green beans or crudités. You would be surprised at just how many restaurants will do this.

- Go for soup! Soups are great as a filler, and many soups, such as vegetable or bean, are high in nutrients. Stay away from cream-based soups; choose broth-based ones instead. Research shows that eating soup will often leave you consuming fewer calories overall at the meal.

- Ask for lemon for your water and drink at least a glass before you begin eating. If you prefer herbal or green tea, have that instead.

- Skip at least the first alcoholic beverage. If you do choose to indulge, aim for a high-ORAC drink. Remember, alcohol lowers your defenses, making it easier to inadvertently overconsume food. Sip, don't chug, that wine!

- If you opt for dessert, remember, go ORAC! Every food you consume is an opportunity to consume nutrients. Go for mixed berries, or tea or a cappuccino made with fat-free milk.

After you've eaten

- Try to allow yourself time to digest your food before going to bed. Going to bed with a full stomach often makes you extra hungry in the morning. Plus, your body does not digest food as well if you go to sleep immediately after a meal.

- Walk home from the restaurant or take a stroll around your neighborhood. A refreshing walk is a good way to help burn a few extra calories, but the real benefit may be how good it can be for your mind.

O_2 on the run

Even at fast-food restaurants, you can find a few calorie-controlled, high-ORAC foods. Here are a few of my favorite on-the-run ORAC meals.

Subway

6-inch Oven Roasted Chicken Breast on Whole Wheat (You can also order this meal as a salad with no bread.)

Pizza Hut

2 slices 12-inch Diced Red Tomato, Mushroom, and Jalapeño Fit 'N Delicious pizza

2 slices 12-inch Green Pepper, Red Onion, and Diced Tomato Fit 'N Delicious pizza

McDonald's

Premium Southwest Salad with Grilled Chicken (Save 35 calories by taking out the tortilla strips, and use the Newman's Own Low Fat Balsamic Vinaigrette for 40 calories.)

Fruit 'N' Yogurt Parfait (without granola) as a snack

Taco Bell

Fresco Bean Burrito

Starbucks

Classic Salad

Oatmeal (Add nuts *or* fruit.)

Grande Green tea skim latte

Coffee with fat-free milk or soy milk, or skim latte (Remember, coffee is the number-one way most Americans consume antioxidants.)

California Pizza Kitchen (½ order)
Moroccan Chicken Salad (skip the dressing and use vinegar)

Chili's
Guiltless Cedar Plank Tilapia

Outback Steakhouse
Grilled Scallops with fresh seasonal veggies

Tony Roma's
Grilled Mahimahi with seared green beans (ask for steamed)

O₂ for life!

You now should be eating in a way that seems livable—for life! To make your diet even more decadent, you can now incorporate one more *conscious indulgence* per week. Be sure to keep those ORAC points high by including one more fruit per day.

What about those times you are left stranded with no high-ORAC choices? When a cream-based pasta dish looks healthy compared to the rest of the menu? Here are a few simple steps to help you through these diet roadblocks:

Use your DIY building blocks to devise the best possible meal when your options are not the best. Let's say that for veggies you may have only the choice of iceberg lettuce or creamed spinach, and your protein choice may be one fatty meat versus another. In this case, use the portion guidelines I have given you and remember your HQ. If you listen to your HQ and *stop* when you are satisfied, you will never overconsume dramatically.

To make up for a low-ORAC meal? The next day, have a couple of O₂ shots, drink an extra cup of green tea, and choose foods high on the ORAC points list; you will most likely average out to 30,000 points for the 2 days. Most important, remember that every meal is an individual opportunity to eat well! Take each meal one at a time and do not let one "bad" meal throw you off. Every meal is a Monday morning—a new time to feed your body the best possible foods. For more O₂ for Life strategies, see my Q&A on page 183.

How to Eat O₂ on the Go

Meal	ORAC Points
Breakfast	
Instant oatmeal	600
1 c fat-free milk	—
8 pecan halves (preportioned in bag to go)	2,500
1 tsp cinnamon (It's easy to carry cinnamon in your bag or keep it in your desk drawer.)	7,000
1 c green tea (Again, keep those tea bags in your bag, glove compartment, desk drawer, wherever.)	3,000
1 c water with lemon (Use a True Lemon packet to throw in water on the fly.)	400
Snack	
Monterey Farms ArtiHearts (You can eat these right out of the bag. Great when you're on the go!)	7,900
1 c water with lemon (Use a True Lemon packet to throw in water on the fly.)	400
Lunch	
Romaine lettuce (any salad bar has this available, or at home you can use prewashed), sliced red and yellow bell peppers (slice them as soon as you get home from the grocery store so you have them on hand to add to salad!), and grape tomatoes	1,400
4 oz canned tuna	—
2 tsp olive oil, 1 oz lemon juice, and ¼ tsp black pepper	700
1 c water with lemon (Use a True Lemon packet to throw in water on the fly.)	400

(continued)

Meal	ORAC Points
Snack	
1 Gala apple (It's easy enough to carry an apple with you!)	5,200
7 walnuts (I like to portion out peanut butter and carry it with me, but if that's too tough, keeping mini bags of nuts around is the easiest option.)	1,900
1 c green tea	3,000
Dinner	
1 c frozen spinach (Sometimes microwaving veggies is the only way to get them in. Frozen is okay!)	3,600
Free Bird Grilled Chicken Strips (These are precooked. It doesn't get any easier!)	—
1/4 c marinara sauce	450
1 Tbsp Parmesan cheese	—
1 tsp oregano	3,600
(Prepare chicken according to package directions, top with marinara, and bake at 350°F until the cheese melts, or microwave for 10 seconds; sprinkle with oregano.)	
1 c water with lemon (Use a True Lemon packet to throw in water on the fly.)	400
4 c water with lemon additional throughout the day	1,600
TOTAL ORAC POINTS	39,050

APPETIZERS

Spinach and artichoke dip served
with tortilla chips and salsa

Steamed mussels in white wine
or tomato sauce

Crab cakes with fresh Maryland lump crab meat

Tuna tartare served over mixed greens

Artichokes Roman style, baked with olive oil, garlic, and parsley

1.
Check out the appetizers and salads. Here is an opportunity to fill up, and up your ORAC! Yum, that artichoke appetizer sounds delish—but it's way high in calories from fat. Ask that no oil be used in baking, and then add your own portion of 2 teaspoons olive oil.

SALADS

Goat cheese salad of mesclun greens,
tomatoes, pine nuts, and balsamic vinaigrette

House salad with lemon and olive oil dressing

Spinach salad with pears, blue cheese, mushrooms,
onions, bacon, walnuts, and sherry vinaigrette

Salade Niçoise with fresh tuna, black olives, tomatoes,
French beans, potatoes, lemon, and olive oil

2.
Look for lean protein. The salmon looks amazing to me here and could be ordered grilled, but the tuna tartare appetizer may actually be a perfect portion for a meal. Ask how hearty a portion the tuna app is, and check in with your HQ before you decide.

SOUPS

French onion soup

Turkey chili

Chicken soup with carrots, celery, and parsnips

SANDWICHES

Grilled vegetable sandwich with mozzarella and balsamic
vinaigrette on a club roll

Grilled chicken breast with pesto mayonnaise on a club roll

Turkey burger with maple glaze

Hamburger, with or without cheese

ENTRÉES

Roasted chicken with lemon and herbs

Rib eye steak (18 ounces) with mashed potatoes and vegetables

Braised lamb shank with vegetable risotto
and roasted garlic sauce

Seared salmon with whole grain mustard sauce
and sautéed spinach

Shrimp scampi sautéed with garlic and
olive oil and served with spaghetti

3.
Don't be afraid to switch things up. If you've gone for the salmon, ask for it grilled, not seared. And request that the spinach be steamed.

SIDES

French fries

Parmesan mashed potatoes

Sautéed broccoli rabe

Sautéed mixed peppers and onions

4.
Choose a side.
Another opportunity to up your ORAC and keep your hands out of the bread basket. In this case, that spinach accompanying the salmon, coupled with the salad, may be enough veggies for your night. But if you feel like splitting a side dish, order the broccoli rabe and ask that the chef go very light on the oil when sautéing.

DESSERTS

Apple crumb pie

Chocolate soufflé cake

Fresh fruit plate

Assorted cookies

5.
Dessert?
Ask yourself whether you want to make this a *conscious indulgence* night. If the meal was satisfying, how about a cup of mint tea instead?

6.
Drink up!
Every restaurant has water and lemon. Drink it throughout the meal.

Your 6-Step Plan for Choosing a Healthy O₂ Meal

1. Cool beans. Edamame is the perfect side to up your ORAC and provide a little more protein to help provide satiety.

Appetizers

Edamame (steamed soy beans with sea salt)

Tuna Tataki (tuna tartare)

Sake Tataki (salmon tartare)

Shrimp Shumai (steamed shrimp dumplings)

Negimaki (broiled beef with scallion and mushroom)

Rock Shrimp Tempura with wasabi sauce

Miso Eggplant

Vegetable Tempura

Salads

Seaweed Salad with sesame dressing

Green Salad with ginger dressing

Hijiki Salad, black seaweed with mushrooms

2. Choose salad. Instead of the same old green salad, go for the hijiki salad. Hijiki is high in fiber and will help fill you up. However, it is hard to find and may be too daring for some of you. If that's the case, go for the simple green salad and ask for dressing on the side. Use 1 tablespoon.

Soups

Miso Soup

Clear Soup, dashi base with scallion

Seafood Soup

3. Smart soups. If you are in the mood for soup, miso soup is a "freebie." Studies even show that those who eat soup end up eating less at the meal because it helps fill you up.

Sushi/Sashimi

Tuna

Yellow Tail

Salmon

Unagi, eel

Ebi, broiled shrimp

Hotate, sea scallop

Tamago, egg

Crabstick

4. Look for lean protein. If you have not had your fill of salmon then this is an easy place to fill up on some omega-3s. Usually four pieces of sashimi is the perfect portion of protein.

Rolls

California Roll

Spicy Tuna with Tempura Flakes

Spicy Lobster Roll

Shrimp Tempura Roll

Sweet Potato Tempura Roll

Eel Avocado Roll

Spider Roll, soft shell crab, cucumber, and avocado

Cucumber Roll

Salmon Skin Roll

Philadelphia Roll, smoked salmon and cream cheese

**5.
Don't be afraid to switch things up.** If you don't like sashimi because you need a little rice or veggie to flavor it up, ask for hand rolls with no rice and substitute veggies in place of the rice. Most restaurants do this for you no problem!

Entrées

Miso Black Cod

Seafood Cha Soba (stir-fried buckwheat noodles with seafood)

Teriyaki (choice of chicken, beef, tofu, vegetable, or seafood)

Tempura (choice of vegetable, chicken, or shrimp)

Yaki Udon (choice of chicken, beef, vegetable, or seafood)

Sides

White Rice

Brown Rice

Desserts

Banana Tempura

Ice Cream Tempura, green tea, vanilla

Mochi Ice Cream, green tea, vanilla

Almond Cookies

**6.
Drink up!** Is there any better place to up your ORAC with green tea?

Your O₂ Recipes

Breakfast
PHASE II AND BEYOND

Salmon and Feta Omelet with Asparagus

1 omega-3-enriched egg

2 egg whites

$\frac{1}{8}$ teaspoon freshly ground black pepper

$\frac{1}{4}$ teaspoon fresh dill, finely chopped

1 tablespoon garlic-and-herb-flavored feta cheese (such as Athenos)

2 ounces canned wild pink salmon, drained, picked over, and chunked (about $\frac{1}{4}$ cup)

$\frac{1}{4}$ cup chopped and drained canned or steamed asparagus (about 2)

1. Place a small nonstick skillet over medium heat and coat with canola oil cooking spray.
2. In a small bowl, beat the egg, egg whites, black pepper, and dill.
3. Pour the egg mixture into the skillet. Scatter the feta, salmon, and asparagus on top. Cook 2 minutes, or until the edges bubble and the middle is still loose. Flip and cook about 1 minute, then flip again and cook about 1 minute longer, or until the egg is cooked through and no longer runny. Season with salt and freshly ground black pepper to taste.
4. Serve with 1 cup blackberries.

Makes 1 omelet

ORAC Value: 8,500

Veggie and Cheddar Miniquiches

1 tablespoon + 2 teaspoons wheat germ

1 tablespoon ground flaxseed

2 omega-3-enriched eggs

2 egg whites

2 tablespoons fat-free milk

$\frac{1}{2}$ cup fat-free cottage cheese

$\frac{1}{8}$ teaspoon garlic powder

$\frac{1}{4}$ teaspoon freshly ground black pepper

$\frac{1}{4}$ teaspoon finely chopped fresh tarragon

$\frac{1}{4}$ cup shredded reduced-fat Cheddar cheese

1 cup chopped cooked broccoli

$\frac{1}{2}$ cup chopped mushrooms

Parmesan cheese (optional)

1. Preheat the oven to 350°F. Coat a 6-cup nonstick muffin pan with canola oil cooking spray.
2. Combine the wheat germ and flaxseed in a small bowl. Add 1 heaping teaspoon of the mixture to each muffin cup, spreading to coat the bottoms evenly.
3. Whisk the eggs, egg whites, milk, and cottage cheese in a bowl. Add the garlic powder, black pepper, tarragon, and Cheddar cheese and whisk until combined.
4. Stir in the broccoli and mushrooms and divide the mixture among the muffin cups, using $\frac{1}{4}$-cup measures.
5. Bake 30 to 35 minutes on the middle rack in the oven, or until the miniquiches are lightly browned on top and a knife inserted in the center comes out clean. Let them cool in the pan on a rack 5 to 10 minutes; use a knife to loosen the edges from the pan and remove the miniquiches. Serve sprinkled with the Parmesan cheese, if desired.
6. Serve with 1 cup blueberries.

Makes 3 servings (2 miniquiches each)

ORAC Value: 11,000

Green Tea Walnut Loaf

1¼ cups whole grain pastry flour

½ cup turbinado sugar

1 teaspoon baking powder

½ teaspoon baking soda

½ teaspoon salt

½ teaspoon ground cloves

1 teaspoon ground cinnamon

2 egg whites

½ cup fat-free plain yogurt

¼ cup steeped green tea, cooled to room temperature

¼ cup safflower or canola oil

1 teaspoon pure vanilla extract

¾ cup chopped walnuts

1. Preheat the oven to 350°F. Coat an 8" x 4" loaf pan with canola oil cooking spray.
2. Combine the flour, sugar, baking powder, baking soda, salt, cloves, and cinnamon in a large bowl.
3. Whisk the egg whites, yogurt, green tea, oil, and vanilla extract in a small bowl until just combined.
4. Make a well in the center of the flour mixture and add the egg white mixture. Mix until well combined, then evenly fold in the walnuts.
5. Pour the batter into the prepared loaf pan. Bake 40 to 45 minutes on the middle rack in the oven, or until a knife inserted in the center comes out clean.
6. Serve with 1 teaspoon nut butter.

Makes 8 servings

Note: Slice and portion immediately after the bread cools. You can also freeze the portions if you like.

ORAC Value: 2,100

Paradise Smoothie

1 medium ripe peach, sliced

2 tablespoons chopped Hass avocado

$\frac{1}{3}$ cup unsweetened frozen strawberries

$\frac{3}{4}$ cup fat-free plain yogurt

3 tablespoons 100% pomegranate juice

1 teaspoon grapeseed oil

1 teaspoon pure vanilla extract

Place the peach, avocado, strawberries, yogurt, juice, oil, and vanilla extract in a blender. Puree about 15 seconds, or until smooth. Pour into a tall glass and serve.

Makes 1 serving

ORAC Value: 5,300

My Favorite O₂ Food
Katie Lee, author of *The Comfort Table*

I like to mix a teaspoon of cinnamon into my coffee grounds before brewing. The touch of spice adds a subtle hint of flavor, and the exotic aroma creates a magical moment in the rush of a weekday morning.

Caramelized Pear and Pecan French Toast

TOPPING

$\frac{1}{4}$ teaspoon pure vanilla extract

$\frac{1}{3}$ cup peeled and chopped pear

1 tablespoon chopped pecans

$\frac{1}{8}$ teaspoon ground cinnamon

1 teaspoon honey, divided

FRENCH TOAST

1 omega-3-enriched egg

1 tablespoon fat-free milk

$\frac{1}{8}$ teaspoon ground cinnamon

1 slice 100% whole wheat bread

1. Place a nonstick skillet over medium heat and coat with canola oil cooking spray.
2. Combine the vanilla, pear, pecans, $\frac{1}{8}$ teaspoon cinnamon, and $\frac{1}{2}$ teaspoon of the honey in a small bowl and stir to coat. Add the mixture to the skillet and cook, stirring, 3 to 5 minutes, or until lightly browned. Remove from the skillet and set aside. Coat the skillet once more with cooking spray and return to the heat.
3. Beat the egg, milk, and $\frac{1}{8}$ teaspoon cinnamon in a shallow bowl. With a fork, dip the bread into the egg mixture. Flip to coat both sides.
4. Place the bread in the skillet and cook, 1 minute per side, or until the bread is lightly browned and the egg is cooked.
5. Top with the reserved topping and serve drizzled with the remaining $\frac{1}{2}$ teaspoon honey.

Makes 1 serving

ORAC Value: 4,600

Tropical Sunrise Oatmeal

$\frac{1}{3}$ cup cooked rolled oats, prepared with light soy milk

1 tablespoon canned light coconut milk

$\frac{1}{4}$ teaspoon pure vanilla extract

$\frac{1}{8}$ teaspoon ground cinnamon

$\frac{1}{8}$ teaspoon ground nutmeg

$\frac{1}{4}$ cup coarsely chopped ripe mango

1 tablespoon chopped macadamia nuts

$\frac{1}{2}$ teaspoon honey

1. Combine the oats, coconut milk, and vanilla extract in a small bowl. Add the cinnamon and nutmeg and stir to combine.
2. Top with the mango and macadamia nuts and drizzle with honey. Sprinkle with additional cinnamon, if desired.

Makes 1 serving

ORAC Value: 2,000

Banana-Nut Butter Waffle

1 whole grain frozen waffle

2 teaspoons almond, cashew, or peanut butter

$1/4$ cup thinly sliced banana (about $1/3$ banana)

Dash of ground cinnamon

$1/2$ teaspoon honey (optional)

1. Toast the waffle according to the package directions.
2. Spread the almond butter on the waffle and top with the banana. Sprinkle with the cinnamon and lightly drizzle with honey, if using.

Makes 1 serving

ORAC Value: 1,200

Spiced Applesauce Pancake

1 egg white

1 tablespoon fat-free milk or plain light soy milk

1 teaspoon safflower or canola oil

4 tablespoons unsweetened applesauce, divided

2 tablespoons wheat germ

2 tablespoons whole grain pastry flour

$\frac{1}{8}$ teaspoon ground ginger

$\frac{1}{8}$ teaspoon baking powder

$\frac{1}{4}$ teaspoon ground cinnamon, divided

$\frac{1}{2}$ cup fat-free plain yogurt

1. Beat the egg white and milk in a small bowl. Add the oil and 2 tablespoons of the applesauce and stir until just combined.
2. Combine the wheat germ, flour, ginger, baking powder, and $\frac{1}{8}$ teaspoon cinnamon in a medium bowl. Add the egg white mixture and stir until just combined. Let stand.
3. Place a nonstick skillet over medium heat and coat with cooking spray.
4. Reduce the heat to low. Spoon the batter into the skillet, spreading evenly to form a circle. Cook 1 minute 30 seconds, or until the edges bubble slightly. Flip. Cook 1 minute, then flip again and cook 1 minute longer, or until the center is firm.
5. Combine the yogurt, remaining 2 tablespoons applesauce, and remaining $\frac{1}{8}$ teaspoon cinnamon in a small bowl. Serve the pancake topped with the yogurt mixture. Garnish with additional cinnamon, if desired.

Makes 1 pancake

ORAC Value: 3,000

Berry Creamy Quinoa Parfait

$\frac{1}{3}$ cup cooked quinoa

$\frac{1}{2}$ cup fat-free plain yogurt

$\frac{1}{2}$ teaspoon honey (optional)

$\frac{1}{4}$ teaspoon pure vanilla extract

$\frac{1}{8}$ teaspoon ground cinnamon

$\frac{1}{3}$ cup fresh or frozen and thawed blueberries

$\frac{1}{4}$ cup frozen pure unsweetened acai berry puree (such as Sambazon), thawed

2 tablespoons chopped walnuts

1. Mix the quinoa, yogurt, honey (if using), vanilla extract, and cinnamon in a small bowl.
2. Fold the blueberries gently into the acai pulp in another small bowl, stirring to coat.
3. Spoon $\frac{1}{3}$ of the quinoa mixture into a glass, then $\frac{1}{3}$ of the blueberry mixture and $\frac{1}{3}$ of the walnuts. Repeat the layers twice, ending with walnuts on top.

Makes 1 serving

ORAC Value: 9,000

My Favorite O$_2$ Food
Gary Hirshberg, president and CE-Yo, Stonyfield Farm

My favorite source of antioxidants is acai. I love taking Sambazon frozen acai pulp and making smoothies in the morning with our plain Oikos Greek yogurt or with vanilla low-fat yogurt. If you add an organic banana or some frozen organic blueberries and maybe some wheat germ, the smoothie is totally satisfying and filling. In fact, I try to bike to work (28 miles) whenever I can, and I have learned that a smoothie like this can easily give me all the energy I need for the ride.

Very Berry Oat Cake

$\frac{1}{2}$ cup almond meal

$\frac{1}{2}$ cup turbinado sugar

$2\frac{1}{2}$ teaspoons baking powder

$\frac{1}{2}$ teaspoon salt

$1\frac{1}{2}$ cups + 1 tablespoon oat flour

1 omega-3-enriched egg

$\frac{1}{4}$ cup extravirgin olive oil

$\frac{1}{2}$ cup fat-free milk

1 cup frozen blackberries

1 cup frozen raspberries

$\frac{1}{2}$ cup rolled oats

$\frac{3}{4}$ teaspoon ground cinnamon

1 tablespoon honey

1. Preheat the oven to 350°F. Coat a 9" round cake pan with canola oil cooking spray.
2. Combine the almond meal, sugar, baking powder, salt, and $1\frac{1}{2}$ cups of the flour in a large bowl.
3. Whisk the egg, oil, and milk in a small bowl just until combined.
4. Add the egg mixture to the flour mixture and mix well.
5. Toss the blackberries and raspberries with the remaining flour in a medium bowl to coat. Gently fold the berries into the batter and pour into the prepared pan.
6. Combine the oats, cinnamon, and honey in a small bowl. Using clean fingers, sprinkle the honey-oat mixture over the cake batter, loosely covering the surface of the cake.
7. Bake 40 to 45 minutes on the middle rack in the oven, or until a knife inserted in the center comes out clean and the topping is lightly browned. Let cool completely in the pan on a rack before serving.

Makes 8 servings

Note: Slice and portion immediately after the cake cools. You can also freeze the portions if you like.

ORAC Value: 3,400

Fig-Filled Muffins

8 dried Mission figs (about $\frac{1}{2}$ cup)

2 teaspoons finely grated lemon peel, divided

1 cup whole grain pastry flour

$\frac{1}{4}$ cup ground flaxseed

1 teaspoon baking powder

$\frac{1}{2}$ teaspoon salt

1 teaspoon ground cinnamon

1 egg white

$\frac{1}{2}$ cup fat-free or light soy milk

3 tablespoons canola or safflower oil

$\frac{1}{2}$ teaspoon pure vanilla extract

$\frac{1}{4}$ cup honey

3 tablespoons unsweetened applesauce

1. Preheat the oven to 375°F. Line a 6-cup muffin pan or coat it with canola oil cooking spray.
2. In a blender, puree the figs and 1 teaspoon of the lemon peel into a chunky paste, about 10 seconds, using a spatula to scrape down the sides halfway through. Set aside.
3. Combine the flour, flaxseed, baking powder, salt, cinnamon, and remaining teaspoon lemon peel in a large bowl.
4. Whisk the egg white, milk, oil, and vanilla extract in a small bowl. Whisk in the honey and applesauce until well combined. Add the egg mixture to the flour mixture and mix well.
5. Fill the prepared muffin cups just below halfway, using scant $\frac{1}{8}$-cup measures. Add a rounded teaspoonful of the reserved fig mixture to the center of each muffin cup. Divide the remaining batter among the muffin cups, covering the fig mixture completely.
6. Bake 23 to 25 minutes on the middle rack in the oven, or until lightly browned on top and a knife inserted in the center about halfway through comes out clean. Let cool in the pan 5 to 10 minutes before turning out onto a rack.
7. Serve with $\frac{1}{4}$ cup fat-free cottage cheese.

Makes 6 muffins

ORAC Value: 3,200

Chocolate-Cherry Buttermilk Scones

1 cup white whole wheat flour

1 cup almond meal

$\frac{1}{3}$ cup turbinado sugar

2 teaspoons baking powder

$\frac{1}{2}$ teaspoon baking soda

$\frac{1}{2}$ teaspoon salt

$\frac{1}{2}$ teaspoon ground cardamom

$\frac{1}{2}$ cup light buttermilk + additional for brushing

2 teaspoons almond extract

2 tablespoons safflower oil

$\frac{1}{2}$ cup dark chocolate chips or chunks

$\frac{3}{4}$ cup frozen dark cherries, quartered

1. Preheat the oven to 375°F. Line a baking sheet with parchment paper.
2. Combine the flour, almond meal, sugar, baking powder, baking soda, salt, and cardamom in a large bowl. Add the buttermilk, almond extract, and oil. Mix well, until the dry ingredients are completely incorporated.
3. Using a spatula, fold in the chocolate chips, then very gently fold in the cherries just until combined. Do not overmix.
4. Using generous $\frac{1}{4}$-cup measures, drop the batter about 1" apart onto the prepared baking sheet. Lightly brush the surface of the scones with buttermilk. Bake 18 to 20 minutes, or until the tops are lightly golden brown and firm to the touch.
5. Serve with $\frac{1}{2}$ cup fat-free plain yogurt and $\frac{1}{2}$ teaspoon honey.

Makes 9 scones

ORAC Value: 1,400

Lunch
PHASE II AND BEYOND

Quick Cobb Salad

1 tablespoon freshly squeezed lemon juice

1 teaspoon grapeseed oil

1/4 teaspoon finely chopped fresh dill

2 cups chopped red leaf or romaine lettuce

1/2 cup grape tomatoes, halved

1/4 cup thinly sliced cucumber, quartered

2 tablespoons finely chopped red onion

2 tablespoons chopped avocado

1 tablespoon shelled raw or roasted sunflower seeds

1 tablespoon shredded reduced-fat Cheddar cheese

2 slices (2 ounces) roasted prepackaged or deli-sliced turkey

2 slices (2 ounces) uncured prepackaged or deli-sliced ham

1. Combine the lemon juice, oil, and dill in a small bowl. Season with salt and freshly ground black pepper to taste. Set aside.
2. Toss the lettuce, tomatoes, cucumber, onion, avocado, sunflower seeds, and cheese with the reserved dressing in a medium bowl.
3. Lay 1 slice of the turkey flat on the work surface. Layer the ham slice flat on top, then the remaining turkey and ham slices, and tightly roll up. Slice the meat roll crosswise into thin pinwheels and scatter them on top of the salad.

Makes 1 serving

ORAC Value: 3,200

Deviled Egg Salad "Cups"

2 tablespoons low-fat (2%) plain Greek yogurt

1 teaspoon spicy brown or Dijon mustard

$\frac{1}{4}$ teaspoon ground paprika

$\frac{1}{4}$ teaspoon garlic powder

2 omega-3-enriched hard-boiled eggs, chopped

2 tablespoons finely chopped celery

1 tablespoon finely chopped radish (about 1 medium)

1 teaspoon thinly sliced scallion (green part only)

3 small Bibb or Boston lettuce leaves

1. Combine the yogurt, mustard, paprika, and garlic powder in a medium bowl. Add the eggs, celery, radish, and scallion and gently mix to coat. Season to taste with salt and freshly ground black pepper.
2. Place the lettuce leaves on a plate. Spoon the egg salad into the leaf centers and garnish with paprika.
3. Serve with 1 Red Delicious apple.

Makes 1 serving

ORAC Value: 8,900

Roast Beef Roll-Ups

2 teaspoons balsamic vinegar

1 teaspoon extravirgin olive oil

1 cup baby arugula or baby romaine lettuce

3 thin slices (3 ounces) organic roast beef (such as Applegate Farms)

1 jarred roasted red pepper, cut in 3 pieces crosswise

3 large basil leaves

1 ounce fresh mozzarella cheese, cut in 3 small pieces

1. Combine the vinegar and oil in a small bowl.
2. Make a bed of arugula or romaine on a plate. Lay 1 roast beef slice flat on the work surface and layer 1 piece of roasted pepper, 1 basil leaf, and 1 piece of cheese on one side. Tightly roll up and place, edge side down, on the arugula or lettuce. Repeat with the remaining beef slices, basil, and cheese.
3. Drizzle the vinegar-oil mixture over the beef and greens and garnish with freshly ground black pepper. Serve with 1 Wasa Oats Crispbread.

Makes 1 serving

ORAC Value: 1,200

Black-Eyed Pea Salad with Pesto

$^3/_4$ cup canned black-eyed peas

$^1/_4$ cup coarsely chopped jarred marinated artichoke hearts in oil (about 2 hearts)

$^1/_2$ cup grape tomatoes, halved

2 tablespoons sliced black olives

1 tablespoon prepared pesto (such as Buitoni with Basil) or the pesto in Stuffed Chicken Breast with Lemon-Artichoke Pesto (page 143)

1 teaspoon pine nuts

Toss the black-eyed peas, artichoke hearts, tomatoes, and olives with the pesto in a bowl. Garnish with the pine nuts.

Makes 1 serving

ORAC Value: 9,900

Plum and Pecan Spinach Salad with Pomegranate Dressing

1 tablespoon 100% pomegranate juice

1 teaspoon grapeseed oil

1 teaspoon balsamic vinegar

1 teaspoon finely chopped fresh mint

2 cups baby spinach

1 ripe medium plum, cut into 1" pieces

2 tablespoons (1 ounce) reduced-fat feta cheese

2 tablespoons chopped pecans

1 tablespoon raisins

1 tablespoon finely chopped red onion

1. Combine the pomegranate juice, oil, vinegar, and mint in a small bowl. Set aside.
2. Place the spinach, plum, cheese, pecans, raisins, and onion in a medium bowl; toss with the reserved dressing.

Makes 1 serving

ORAC Value: 11,000

My Favorite O_2 Food
Irwin Simon, CEO, The Hain Celestial Group

I love pomegranates. . . . There are a multitude of ways to incorporate them into my diet as either a snack, a drink, a dressing, or even a garnish! Instead of drinking soda, I'll mix club soda and pomegranate juice for a delicious drink. If I'm making a citrus-flavored dressing or marinade, I'll use pomegranate as a substitute for lemon juice. I even use pomegranates as a garnish—not only are they full of flavor, they help add a dash of color and texture to any meal.

Tuna and Chickpea Salad

2 teaspoons red wine vinegar

1 teaspoon extravirgin olive oil

$\frac{1}{2}$ teaspoon minced garlic

$\frac{1}{2}$ cup canned chickpeas

2 ounces canned light tuna in water or olive oil, drained and chunked
  (about $\frac{1}{4}$ cup)

$\frac{1}{4}$ cup canned sliced beets, quartered

2 tablespoons chopped red bell pepper

1 tablespoon finely chopped red onion

$\frac{1}{4}$ cup chopped celery + 2 teaspoons chopped celery leaves

1. Combine the vinegar, oil, and garlic in a small bowl.
2. Toss the vinegar-oil mixture with the chickpeas, tuna, beets, bell pepper, onion, and celery in a medium bowl. Season with salt and freshly ground black pepper to taste.

Makes 1 serving

ORAC Value: 3,000

Dijon Salmon Cakes and Arugula with Lemon-Caper Oil

4 ounces boneless, skinless pink salmon, drained

2 teaspoons minced scallion (green and white parts)

¾ teaspoon lemon peel

3 tablespoons + ½ teaspoon fat-free plain yogurt

2 teaspoons whole grain Dijon mustard, divided

2 teaspoons white horseradish, divided

2 tablespoons wheat germ

3 tablespoons diced celery

½ teaspoon capers, chopped

1 tablespoon freshly squeezed lemon juice

1 teaspoon extravirgin olive oil

1 cup baby arugula

1. Using a fork, combine the salmon, scallion, lemon peel, 3 tablespoons yogurt, 1 teaspoon of the mustard, and 1 teaspoon of the horseradish in a medium bowl. Add the wheat germ and celery and season with salt and freshly ground black pepper. Mix well.
2. Coat a medium nonstick skillet with canola oil cooking spray and place over medium heat about 1 minute. Mix the capers, lemon juice, and oil in a medium bowl. Add the arugula and toss to coat. Transfer to a serving plate, forming a bed of the arugula mixture. Set aside.
3. Divide the salmon mixture into 2 round patties, each ½" thick. Reduce the heat to low and add the patties to the skillet. Cook 2 minutes per side, then flip and cook 1 minute more, or until heated through and lightly browned. Place on top of the reserved arugula mixture.
4. Combine the remaining ½ teaspoon yogurt, 1 teaspoon mustard, and 1 teaspoon horseradish in a small bowl. Spoon on top of the salmon cakes.

Makes 1 serving

ORAC Value: 2,500

Crunchy Chicken Salad Boats

3 tablespoons fat-free plain yogurt

1 teaspoon apple cider vinegar

$\frac{1}{2}$ teaspoon honey

$\frac{1}{4}$ teaspoon grated gingerroot

3 ounces shredded rotisserie chicken breast, skin removed, or cooked chicken breast (about $\frac{3}{4}$ cup)

1 tablespoon + 1 teaspoon chopped walnuts

2 tablespoons finely chopped Granny Smith apple

2 tablespoons quartered red grapes

2 Kirby cucumbers, halved lengthwise

1. Combine the yogurt, vinegar, honey, and gingerroot in a medium bowl.
2. Add the chicken, walnuts, and apple. Mix well. Gently stir in the grapes until just combined.
3. Seed and scoop out some of the flesh from the cucumber halves using a rounded teaspoon or melon baller. Divide the chicken salad among the cucumber boats.

Makes 1 serving

ORAC Value: 4,000

My Favorite O_2 Food
James Joseph, PhD, Tufts University researcher

I eat a variety of foods every day, but blueberries are important, and I love walnuts. God knew what he was doing when he made walnuts! Dark chocolate every day is okay, too.

Tex-Mex Black Bean Soup

¼ cup cubed avocado

¼ cup grape tomatoes, halved

2 teaspoons finely chopped red onion

1 teaspoon chopped cilantro

1 teaspoon freshly squeezed lime juice

1 cup canned Health Valley No-Salt-Added Organic Black Bean Soup

1 ounce shredded rotisserie chicken breast, skin removed (about ¼ cup), or cooked chicken breast

2 tablespoons shredded reduced-fat Cheddar cheese

1. Combine the avocado, tomatoes, red onion, cilantro, and lime juice in a small bowl. Set aside.
2. Stir the soup and chicken in a small saucepan over medium heat. Cook, stirring, 2 minutes. Add the cheese, stirring constantly, and continue to cook until the cheese is melted.
3. Top the soup with the avocado-tomato mixture and serve immediately.

Makes 1 serving

ORAC Value: 16,500

Mediterranean Shrimp Pita

3 tablespoons freshly squeezed lemon juice

2 teaspoons extravirgin olive oil

1 teaspoon chopped garlic

3 jumbo shrimp, peeled and deveined (about 3 ounces)

$\frac{1}{2}$ cup baby arugula

1 tablespoon chopped oil-packed sun-dried tomato halves (about 2)

$\frac{1}{4}$ teaspoon dried basil

$\frac{1}{4}$ teaspoon dried parsley

2 tablespoons hummus

1 mini whole wheat pita (such as Thomas' Sahara)

1. Combine the lemon juice, oil, and garlic in a small bowl. Transfer the mixture to a zipper-lock bag and add the shrimp, tossing to coat. Refrigerate 15 minutes.
2. Coat a nonstick grill pan with canola oil cooking spray. Preheat over medium-high heat. Toss the arugula and tomatoes in a small bowl.
3. Remove the shrimp from the marinade. Sprinkle the basil and parsley on both sides and season with salt and freshly ground black pepper. Cook 2 minutes per side, or until opaque throughout, flipping halfway through. Let cool 1 to 2 minutes and cut into $\frac{1}{2}$" pieces.
4. Spread the hummus inside the pita. Fill with the arugula-tomato mixture, then add the shrimp.

Makes 1 serving

ORAC Value: 1,600

Open-Faced Turkey Melt with Cranberry-Cabbage Slaw

½ cup shredded red cabbage

½ teaspoon honey

½ teaspoon red wine vinegar

1 tablespoon sweetened dried cranberries

½ teaspoon finely chopped marjoram or ¼ teaspoon dried

2 teaspoons whole grain Dijon mustard, divided

1 slice oat nut bread

2 slices (2 ounces) roasted prepackaged or deli-sliced turkey (such as Applegate Farms)

1 slice (1 ounce) reduced-fat Swiss cheese (such as Alpine Lace)

1. Line a broiler rack with foil and place it about 4" from the heat. Preheat the broiler.
2. Combine the cabbage, honey, vinegar, cranberries, marjoram, and 1 teaspoon of the mustard in a small bowl.
3. Spread the remaining 1 teaspoon mustard on the bread. Layer on the turkey, then the cabbage mixture, and place the cheese on top. Broil 3 minutes, or until the cheese is melted and bubbly.

Makes 1 serving

ORAC Value: 4,200

Greek Chicken Stack
with Herbed Yogurt Spread

$1/3$ cup low-fat (2%) Greek yogurt

1 teaspoon minced garlic

$3/4$ teaspoon chopped fresh parsley

$1/2$ teaspoon fresh thyme

$1/4$ teaspoon dried oregano

4 ounces boneless, skinless chicken breast

1 slice pumpernickel bread

1 leaf red leaf lettuce

4 thin slices cucumber

1 thin slice red onion

1. Combine the yogurt, garlic, parsley, thyme, and oregano in a shallow bowl. Season with salt and freshly ground black pepper to taste. Reserve 2 table-spoons of the yogurt-herb mixture, cover with plastic wrap, and refrigerate.
2. In a bowl, coat the chicken on all sides with the remaining yogurt-herb mixture. Cover with plastic wrap and refrigerate 15 minutes.
3. Coat a nonstick grill pan with canola oil cooking spray and preheat over medium-high heat. Cook the chicken about 6 minutes per side, or until cooked through.
4. Spread 1 tablespoon of the reserved yogurt-herb mixture on the bread. Place the lettuce and chicken on top. Spread the remaining yogurt-herb mixture over the chicken and top with the cucumber and onion.

Makes 1 serving

ORAC Value: 2,300

My Favorite O$_2$ Food
Gail Simmons,
Food & Wine and *Bravo*'s *Top Chef*

My favorite healthy sources of antioxidants, often overlooked, are ground spices and fresh herbs. I always keep fresh herbs on hand, and I use them as often as possible in salads, dressings, and sauces, or to add to grilled, roasted, or sautéed meats. In a pinch, dried herbs will work, too!

Dinner
PHASE II AND BEYOND

Salmon with Raspberry-Balsamic Glaze

6 fresh raspberries

2 tablespoons balsamic vinegar

1 teaspoon freshly squeezed orange juice

$\frac{1}{4}$ teaspoon orange peel

$\frac{1}{2}$ teaspoon honey

Splash of red wine (about 1 teaspoon)

4 ounces skinless salmon fillet, preferably wild (about $\frac{3}{4}$" thick)

1. Mash the raspberries and vinegar with a fork in a small bowl. Stir in the orange juice, orange peel, honey, and wine until combined. Set aside.
2. Coat a nonstick skillet with canola oil cooking spray and place over medium heat. Cook the salmon about 4 minutes per side, or until the fish is cooked through. Set aside. Remove the skillet from the heat and carefully wipe away any liquid with a paper towel.
3. Return the skillet to medium heat and add the reserved raspberry mixture. Stirring constantly, cook 2 minutes, or until just thickened.
4. Pour the sauce over the salmon and serve with asparagus on the side.

Makes 1 serving

ORAC Value: 4,700

Italian Pork Sliders

4 ounces ground pork

2 tablespoons chopped onion

1 teaspoon minced garlic

1 tablespoon chopped parsley

$\frac{1}{4}$ teaspoon dried oregano

3 tablespoons jarred tomato sauce

1 tablespoon part-skim mozzarella cheese

1. Combine the pork, onion, garlic, parsley, and oregano in a medium bowl. Season with salt and freshly ground black pepper. Divide and form into 3 patties and flatten to about $\frac{1}{2}$" thick.
2. Coat a nonstick skillet with canola oil cooking spray and place the skillet over medium heat. Reduce the heat to low. Add the patties and cook 4 to 5 minutes, flip, and cook 4 more minutes.
3. Flip the patties once more and spoon 1 tablespoon tomato sauce on top of each patty. Top each with 1 teaspoon of the cheese. Cover and cook about 2 more minutes, or until the cheese melts.
4. Serve with steamed broccoli.

Makes 1 serving

ORAC Value: 5,300

Scallop Chowder

1 baby Red Bliss potato (1 to 2 ounces)

1 teaspoon safflower or canola oil

$\frac{1}{4}$ cup chopped leeks, white and pale green parts

$\frac{1}{4}$ cup chopped kale

1 ounce chopped deli ham (about 1 slice)

$\frac{3}{4}$ cup fat-free milk

$\frac{1}{2}$ teaspoon chopped thyme

$\frac{1}{2}$ teaspoon chopped fresh parsley

$\frac{1}{4}$ cup frozen sweet corn

2 ounces bay scallops (about 6), quartered

1. Steam or microwave the potato until it is easily pierced with a fork but still firm. Let cool to room temperature and grate into ribbons.
2. Heat the oil in a small saucepan over medium heat. Add the leeks and kale and cook, stirring constantly, for 2 minutes. Add the ham and cook, stirring, 1 more minute, until the mixture is fragrant and the leeks are softened.
3. Stir in the milk, thyme, parsley, and corn and bring to a simmer, about 5 minutes. Add the scallops and cook, stirring, 2 to 3 minutes more, or until the scallops are opaque and cooked through. Season to taste with salt and freshly ground black pepper. Garnish with nutmeg, if desired.

Makes 1 serving

ORAC Value: 2,700

Chicken Mole

2 teaspoons extravirgin olive oil

1/4 cup chopped onion

1/4 cup chopped poblano or green bell pepper

1 teaspoon coarsely chopped garlic

1/2 cup canned diced tomatoes with juice

1/2 cup fat-free chicken broth

4 ounces boneless, skinless chicken breast

1/4 teaspoon cumin

1 teaspoon chopped bittersweet or semisweet dark chocolate

1 teaspoon chopped cilantro

1. Heat the oil in a small saucepan over medium heat for about 1 minute. Reduce the heat to low and cook the onion, poblano or bell pepper, and garlic 2 to 3 minutes, or until the onion is golden and the pepper is slightly softened.
2. Stir in the tomatoes and chicken broth and bring to a simmer. Rub the chicken on all sides with the cumin and season with salt and freshly ground black pepper. Add the chicken to the pan, spooning some of the broth mixture on top. Cover and simmer 8 to 10 minutes.
3. Turn off the heat. Transfer the chicken to a plate, reserving the broth mixture in the pan. Add the chocolate and cilantro to the broth and stir 15 to 30 seconds, until the chocolate is melted and the sauce thickens.
4. Top the chicken with the sauce and garnish with additional cilantro, if desired. Serve with 1/2 cup canned or frozen sweet corn on the side.

Makes 1 serving

ORAC Value: 7,700

Sage-Crusted Chicken Tenders and Crispy Kale "Chips"

CHICKEN TENDERS

1 egg white

1 tablespoon sesame seeds

1 tablespoon shelled roasted sunflower seeds, finely chopped

$3/4$ teaspoon finely chopped sage

$1/8$ teaspoon freshly ground black pepper

2 boneless, skinless chicken tenders (2 ounces each)

1 tablespoon spicy brown mustard

1 teaspoon honey

KALE "CHIPS"

$1\frac{1}{2}$ cups packed kale cut into $1\frac{1}{2}$" pieces

1 teaspoon minced garlic

1 teaspoon extravirgin olive oil

$1/2$ teaspoon sesame seeds

1. Preheat the oven to 400°F. Coat a baking sheet with canola oil cooking spray.
2. Place the egg white in a shallow bowl. Combine the sesame seeds, sunflower seeds, sage, and black pepper in another small bowl.
3. Using a fork, dip the tenders in the egg white to coat both sides, then dip in the sesame seed mixture, coating both sides. Transfer to one half of the

---

My Favorite O₂ Food
Shane Philip Coffey, executive chef, LuLu Wilson restaurant, Aspen, Colorado

I make a kale salad with currants, Parmesan, pine nuts, lemon, and olive oil. It's proof that something so good for you can be delicious, too! I strongly believe that your body craves what it needs. I guess that's why so many people are addicted to this salad.

baking sheet and mist the surface of the chicken with cooking spray. Flip the tenders with the fork and mist the other side.

4. Combine the kale, garlic, oil, and sesame seeds in a small bowl, tossing to coat. Season with salt and freshly ground black pepper. Transfer to the other half of the baking sheet. (Note: The kale does not need to be in a single layer.)

5. Bake 15 to 17 minutes, or until the chicken is cooked through and the kale is crisp and edges are browned. Flip the tenders and toss the kale halfway through the cooking time.

6. Combine the mustard and honey in a small bowl and serve as a dipping sauce for the tenders.

Makes 1 serving

ORAC Value: 4,400

Chili-Lime Tilapia
with Mango-Avocado Salsa

4 ounces skinless tilapia fillet, about ¼" thick

¼ teaspoon chili powder

Juice of ½ lime plus 2 teaspoons freshly squeezed

¼ cup chopped mango

2 tablespoons cubed avocado

1 tablespoon minced red onion

1 tablespoon diced red bell pepper

1 teaspoon finely chopped cilantro

1 teaspoon finely chopped jalapeño chile pepper (optional)

1. Preheat the oven to 350°F. Coat a glass baking dish with canola oil cooking spray.
2. Rub the fish on all sides with the chili powder. Place in the prepared baking dish, sprinkle with lime juice, and season with salt and freshly ground black pepper. Cover with plastic wrap and refrigerate 15 minutes.
3. Combine the mango, avocado, onion, bell pepper, cilantro, and jalapeño pepper (if using) in a small bowl. Add the 2 teaspoons lime juice and toss well to coat. Let stand.
4. Remove the plastic wrap from the baking dish and bake the fish 15 to 20 minutes, or until the fish is opaque and cooked through. Serve topped with the reserved salsa.

Makes 1 serving

ORAC Value: 1,800

Salsa Chili

2 teaspoons extravirgin olive oil

1 teaspoon finely chopped garlic

3 ounces lean ground turkey

$\frac{1}{4}$ teaspoon ground cumin

$\frac{1}{4}$ teaspoon chili powder

$\frac{1}{2}$ cup jarred chunky red salsa

$1\frac{1}{2}$ teaspoons coarsely chopped roasted cashews

$\frac{1}{4}$ cup canned red kidney beans, rinsed and drained

1. Heat the oil in a small saucepan over medium heat. Reduce the heat to low and add the garlic and turkey. Cook about 3 minutes, stirring constantly to break up the meat and prevent sticking, until the meat is no longer pink.
2. Add the cumin, chili powder, salsa, and cashews, stirring to combine. Cook 1 minute. Stir in the beans and continue cooking 1 more minute, or until heated through.

Makes 1 serving

ORAC Value: 6,100

My Favorite O_2 Food
Curtis Stone, resident chef, NBC's *The Biggest Loser,* and author, *Relaxed Cooking with Curtis Stone*

I love keeping red beans in the cupboard. Not only are they delicious, but they're also packed with antioxidants. They are so versatile, and they look beautiful in whatever you put them in, whether it's a salad or a soup.

Flank Steak with Chimichurri Sauce and Mashed Cauliflower

STEAK AND CHIMICHURRI

4 ounces flank steak

1/8 teaspoon ancho chile powder

1/8 teaspoon sea salt

1/4 teaspoon freshly ground black pepper, divided

1 teaspoon minced garlic

1 teaspoon freshly squeezed lemon juice

1 teaspoon red wine vinegar

2 teaspoons extravirgin olive oil

1/8 teaspoon ground cumin

2 teaspoons finely chopped mint

2 teaspoons finely chopped cilantro

2 teaspoons finely chopped flat-leaf parsley

MASHED CAULIFLOWER

1 cup hot cooked cauliflower florets

1/4 cup fat-free milk, at room temperature

1/4 teaspoon thinly sliced chives

1/4 teaspoon garlic powder

1. Line a broiler rack with foil and place it about 4" from the heat. Preheat the broiler.
2. Rub the flank steak on both sides with the chile powder, salt, and 1/8 teaspoon of the black pepper. Let stand 5 to 10 minutes.
3. Using a fork, combine the garlic, lemon juice, vinegar, oil, and cumin in a small bowl. Add the mint, cilantro, and parsley, the remaining 1/8 teaspoon black pepper, and a dash of salt. Stir until very well combined. Set the sauce aside to let the flavors meld.
4. Place the steak on the prepared rack and broil about 4 minutes per side, or until a thermometer inserted in the center reads 160°F for medium. Let the steak stand 5 minutes before slicing.

5. Place the cauliflower in a blender or a mini food processor fitted with a metal blade. Combine the milk, chives, and garlic powder in a small bowl. Add the milk mixture to the blender and puree about 15 seconds, scraping down the sides with a small spatula halfway through. Season to taste with salt and freshly ground black pepper.
6. Stir and spoon the reserved herb mixture over the steak and serve immediately with the cauliflower.

Makes 1 serving

ORAC Value: 1,900

My Favorite O₂ Food
Chef Spike, top chef and owner, Good Stuff Eatery, Washington, DC

One of the burgers on my menu at Good Stuff Eatery is a free-range turkey burger. We make it with mango chutney, green apples, and a little bit of hot sauce, and we melt Muenster cheese all over it. We finish off with some guacamole and serve it between two pieces of multigrain toasted bun . . . so-o-o delicious. We made this for Michelle Obama at the Easter egg roll at the White House. It's a great way to have your burger but in a healthy, nutrient-rich, and unexpected way.

Sesame Tuna with Jicama-Cabbage Slaw

$\frac{1}{2}$ teaspoon soy sauce

$\frac{1}{2}$ teaspoon rice vinegar (optional)

$\frac{1}{8}$ teaspoon freshly ground black pepper

1 teaspoon toasted sesame oil, divided

$\frac{1}{2}$ cup shredded red cabbage

$\frac{1}{4}$ cup peeled and grated jicama

$\frac{1}{4}$ cup canned mandarin orange segments in light syrup, drained and halved crosswise

2 tablespoons finely chopped red bell pepper

1 teaspoon finely minced scallion (green parts only)

$\frac{1}{4}$ teaspoon black sesame seeds

3 to 4 ounces sushi grade tuna steak, about $\frac{3}{4}$" thick

1. Combine the soy sauce, vinegar (if using), black pepper, and $\frac{1}{2}$ teaspoon of the oil in a small bowl. Add the cabbage, jicama, oranges, bell pepper, scallion, and sesame seeds. Stir to combine and set aside.
2. Preheat a nonstick grill pan over high heat. Rub the tuna on both sides with the remaining $\frac{1}{2}$ teaspoon oil.
3. Cook the tuna 3 to 4 minutes on each side for medium. Remove to a cutting board and thinly slice against the grain.
4. Place a bed of jicama slaw on a serving plate. Top with the tuna and serve immediately.

Makes 1 serving

ORAC Value: 2,400

Stuffed Chicken Breast with Lemon-Artichoke Pesto

¼ cup tightly packed fresh basil leaves

¼ cup jarred marinated artichoke hearts packed in oil, quartered (reserve 1½ teaspoons oil)

½ teaspoon chopped garlic

1 teaspoon lemon juice

¼ teaspoon lemon peel

2 teaspoons chopped walnuts

⅜ teaspoon freshly ground black pepper, divided

5 ounces boneless, skinless chicken breast (½" to ¾" thick)

1 teaspoon extravirgin olive oil

1 tablespoon grated Parmesan cheese

1. Combine the basil, artichokes and oil, garlic, and lemon juice in a blender or mini food processor fitted with a metal blade and process 10 seconds, scraping down the sides halfway through. Add the lemon peel, walnuts, and ⅛ teaspoon of the black pepper. Pulse 10 more seconds, scraping the sides halfway through.
2. Place the chicken breast with its tip toward you and its thickest side closest to your cutting hand. Place your opposite hand on top of the breast. Hold the knife parallel to the cutting surface and slice horizontally, nearly all the way through, leaving the opposite end connected. Spread the top half of the breast open.
3. Place 2 tablespoons of the artichoke mixture in the center of the bottom chicken half and spread the mixture almost to the edges to cover, leaving about a ¼" edge. Fold the opposite breast half over the pesto to cover.
4. Heat the oil in a nonstick skillet over medium heat. Combine the cheese and the remaining ¼ teaspoon black pepper in a small bowl and rub on both sides of the chicken to coat.
5. Cook 4 minutes per side or until the chicken is cooked through. (Note: If the breast is thick, turn to cook all four sides to ensure doneness.) Mix the remaining pesto with a side of steamed green beans, if desired.

Makes 1 serving

ORAC Value: 6,700

Chickpea and Cauliflower Curry

1 teaspoon grapeseed oil

¼ cup coarsely chopped onion

½ cup water

½ cup canned chickpeas, rinsed and drained

½ cup coarsely chopped cauliflower florets

¼ cup baby carrots, cut into rounds

1 tablespoon dried currants or raisins

¼ teaspoon ground cinnamon

¼ teaspoon curry powder

⅛ teaspoon ground turmeric

1 tablespoon light unsweetened coconut milk

2 tablespoons fat-free plain Greek yogurt

1. Heat the oil in a small saucepan over medium heat for about 1 minute. Add the onion and cook about 1 minute, or until softened. Reduce the heat to low. Add the water, chickpeas, cauliflower, carrots, currants, cinnamon, curry powder, turmeric, and coconut milk. Stir to combine.
2. Cover and simmer, stirring occasionally, 8 to 10 minutes, or until the cauliflower is soft and the liquid is mostly absorbed.
3. Season with salt and freshly ground black pepper to taste. Serve topped with yogurt and garnish with additional cinnamon, if desired.

Makes 1 serving

ORAC Value: 4,900 with currants, 4,600 with raisins

Spinach, Bok Choy, and Tofu Stir-Fry

1 tablespoon chunky natural peanut butter

½ teaspoon rice vinegar or honey

¼ teaspoon soy sauce

1 tablespoon water

½ teaspoon minced garlic

¼ teaspoon finely grated gingerroot

¼ teaspoon red pepper flakes

1 teaspoon safflower oil

½ cup trimmed and thinly sliced bok choy ribs and leaves

½ cup tofu, cut into ½" cubes

1 cup baby spinach leaves

¼ cup thinly sliced red bell pepper

¼ cup sliced button mushrooms

1 teaspoon thinly sliced scallion

1. Combine the peanut butter, rice vinegar or honey, soy sauce, and water in a small bowl. Add the garlic, gingerroot, and red pepper flakes. Stir to combine and set aside.
2. Heat the oil in a nonstick skillet over medium heat. Separate the bok choy ribs from the leaves. Place the tofu in a single layer in the skillet and add the bok choy ribs. Cook 2 to 3 minutes, then flip the tofu and cook 3 more minutes, stirring to brown all sides of the tofu.
3. Add the reserved bok choy leaves, spinach, bell pepper, mushrooms, and scallion. Stir in the reserved peanut butter mixture and cook, stirring, 3 more minutes, or until the spinach wilts and the peppers are slightly softened.

Makes 1 serving

ORAC Value: 1,500

Blackberry-Thyme Margarita

Adapted from www.Epicurious.com

16 large fresh blackberries, divided

4 small fresh thyme sprigs, divided

6 tablespoons 100% blue agave silver tequila

$\frac{1}{4}$ cup simple syrup

3 tablespoons freshly squeezed lime juice

1 tablespoon Cointreau or other orange liqueur

2 cups ice cubes, divided

$\frac{1}{4}$ cup chilled sparkling wine

Place 14 of the blackberries and 2 of the thyme sprigs in a medium bowl. With the back of a wooden spoon, press firmly on the solids until mashed. Mix in the tequila, simple syrup, lime juice, and liqueur, then add 1 cup of the ice. Stir to blend well. Strain into a large glass measuring cup. Mix in the sparkling wine. Divide the remaining ice between 2 tall glasses. Pour the margarita mixture over the ice. Garnish each drink with 1 blackberry and 1 thyme sprig.

Makes 2 servings

ORAC Value: 4,320

My Favorite O$_2$ Food
Michele Promaulayko, editor-in-chief, *Women's Health* magazine

At *Women's Health*, we believe that the occasional indulgence is a well-deserved reward for making smart food choices the majority of the time. And if you can work some nutritional benefits into that treat, all the better! One of my favorites: a blackberry-thyme margarita, which qualifies as an antioxidant cocktail, thanks to the blackberries and thyme. Pretty amazing, right?

6

The Outside In:

Beauty Food Fixes
That Pamper

When I talk about beauty foods, I am not simply referring to foods that help you look great from the inside out. I'm referring to foods that are nutritious even when you put them directly *on* your skin. In some cases, topical application is one of the best ways to absorb nutrients. It's true—the same yogurt that is so healthy for your bones and digestive system also makes a great base for your facials!

In recent years, researchers have made big strides in understanding the way the body absorbs chemicals topically—that's why you've heard so much about medicated skin patches for everything from birth control to motion sickness. As we're discovering which kinds of drugs can best be absorbed through the skin, we're also learning tons about how *nutrients* penetrate the skin.

In terms of antioxidants, retinoids have gotten most of the attention since they burst onto the skin care scene back in the 1980s. There are plenty of variations of these vitamin A–derived products on the market, and many dermatologists suggest that adults should start using retinoids daily while they are still in their twenties both to prevent the oxidative damage that comes from the sun and to repair damage that's already happened.

Retinoids aren't the only skin-friendly antioxidants, however. Your epidermis also loves to drink up vitamin C, vitamin E, and ferulic acid (found in wheat bran). All of these—as well as many other micronutrients—keep your skin soft, smooth, and younger looking.

Researchers and cosmetic executives have spent thousands of hours debating what form these compounds should be in for the best absorption. Some types are less stable and begin to deteriorate as soon as they are exposed to air.

But why limit the conversation about absorption to labs and test tubes when you can whip up small batches of these beauty wonders in your own kitchen? These beauty foods are for days when you're feeling like you need a girls' night in or when you've got leftover foods you don't want to waste—Cleopatra bathed in yogurt, after all! An extra bonus: Because you make these potions and lotions yourself, they don't contain the preservatives that irritate some people's skin.

Your O$_2$ Breakthrough:
Don't forget—beauty foods work inside out, too!

As you're pampering your skin with these fun recipes, it doesn't hurt to remind yourself that on the O$_2$ Diet, every meal is a gift to your skin. Not only are all the antioxidants you're eating boosting the ways vitamins A, C, and E can help your skin fight off wrinkles and sun damage as well as renew itself at a healthy pace, but you're also eating plenty of foods that are:

Anti-inflammatory, like fish with omega-3s

Antimicrobial, like the honey you drizzle on your oatmeal at breakfast

Fiber rich, like the apple you have during your coffee break

Hydrating, like that beautiful salad you made last night

These are my favorite recipes for cleansers. Just mix the ingredients together until smooth, then enjoy!

Pink Dairy Cleanser

Milk, yogurt, and sour cream contain lactic acid, which gently exfoliates skin and stimulates collagen, the protein that keeps skin firm and supple. The pink grapefruit pulp in this cleanser protects skin from sun damage and the formation of free radicals.

  2 teaspoons milk

  2 teaspoons pink grapefruit juice, with pulp

  2 teaspoons Greek plain yogurt or sour cream

Sweet Honey Tea Cleanser

Compounds found in honey give it a protective antibacterial activity that can help skin heal faster, and green tea extracts decrease the dangerous effects of sunlight exposure.

  $1/2$ teaspoon honey

  2 teaspoons yogurt

  2 teaspoons brewed green tea or white tea

Blueberry Cream Cleanser

The anthocyanins and other antioxidants in blueberries can be absorbed topically, too. Here they combine with the wrinkle-reducing properties of sour cream.

  $1/8$ cup sour cream

  1 teaspoon brewed green tea

  2 blueberries, mashed

Banana Grape Cleanser

Grape skins contain resveratrol, which helps to protect against inflammation and ultraviolet (UV) light damage. The banana gives this cleanser a great texture and supplies additional antioxidants.

  $1/4$ cup banana

  2 grapes, mashed in a food processor

  $1/2$ teaspoon grapeseed oil

scrubs

For days when skin needs a deeper cleaning, I love to use simple scrubs like these. Simply mix ingredients unless otherwise noted.

Apricot Raspberry Exfoliant

Apricot, chopped fine, acts as an exfoliant to remove dead skin, while the antioxidant properties in the raspberry and its tiny seeds nourish the skin.

   $\frac{1}{4}$ cup yogurt

   1 teaspoon dried apricot, chopped fine

   2 raspberries, mashed

Blueberry Almond Scrub

Besides containing polyphenols, blueberries are high in vitamin C, a treat for thirsty skin. They also provide an antioxidant against skin aging.

   $\frac{1}{4}$ cup plain Greek yogurt

   7 almonds, finely chopped

   7 blueberries, mashed

Caffeinated Yogurt Skin Exhilarator

Coffee, another great exfoliant, has the additional benefit of caffeine, which has been shown to improve fine lines, wrinkles, and discoloration of the skin and to reduce swelling.

   $\frac{1}{4}$ cup plain Greek yogurt

   2 teaspoons ground coffee

Go Green Face Scrub

In this scrub, parsley contains vitamin C for antioxidant protection, and the coarse salt removes the dull outer layer of skin to reveal the younger-looking layers underneath. But the real magic comes from the deep-penetrating avocado oil, which boosts the amount of collagen in your skin. This beauty fix is great for people with mature, sun-damaged, or dehydrated skin. Blend in a food processor for 20 seconds.

1/4 cup avocado

1 teaspoon parsley

2 tablespoons kosher salt

Banana Bread Booster

The almond oil penetrates the skin, slowing down the photoaging process, while the oats exfoliate and soothe inflammation and redness.

1/4 cup banana

7 almonds, sliced or chopped

1/2 teaspoon almond oil

2 teaspoons oats

masks

Once or twice a week, baby your skin with a more intensive treatment that will allow your body to soak in some antioxidants through your skin. Simply mix ingredients (unless otherwise noted), smooth the mixture onto cleansed skin, and put your feet up, taking 15 minutes just to relax.

Honey Oat Facial Mask

The soothing properties of all three ingredients will leave you with a cool, calm glow.

1/4 cup yogurt

3 teaspoons steel-cut oats

1/2 teaspoon honey

Light and Dark Creamed Mask

Forget those stories about chocolate being bad for your skin. Packed with phenols and flavonoids, it softens and smooths.

¼ cup yogurt

1 teaspoon dark chocolate shavings

Tropical Skin Rejuvenator

Mango, full of carotenoids that protect the skin against the formation of free radicals, and papaya, with its skin-soothing enzymes, provide double protection against oxidative damage. And coconut oil is a safe, soothing moisturizer, especially good for rough, dry, or itchy skin. Puree in a food processor until smooth:

⅛ cup ripe mango

⅛ cup ripe papaya

½ teaspoon coconut oil

Calming Skin Mask

Beans provide B vitamins, which protect the skin from the sun and help diminish the signs of wrinkles. Maitake mushrooms may help treat rosacea and redness. Puree in a food processor until smooth.

¼ cup white beans

2 teaspoons maitake mushrooms

Your O$_2$ Breakthrough:
More tea!

Here's the most beautiful reason of all to try some tea: A study from Dartmouth Medical School finds that regular tea drinkers are less likely to get *both* basal cell and squamous cell skin cancer.[2]

Soothing Green and White Mask

Cool as a cucumber? Yep—for the same reasons that cucumber slices feel so refreshing on puffy eyes, this mask soothes redness and inflammation all over, making your skin positively serene. Puree in a food processor until smooth.

$1/4$ cup white beans

5 cucumber slices

Carotenoid Protective Mask

Sweet potatoes and carrots both contain carotenoids, which protect the skin from sun damage and free radicals. The creamy yogurt base makes skin feel firmer. Blend in a food processor for 20 seconds.

$1/4$ peeled sweet potato, baked or microwaved until soft

1 teaspoon thinly sliced carrots

1 teaspoon yogurt

7

The Best
(and Worst)
Things to Eat

For someone who loves to cook and *eat* as much as I do, coming up with a list of "best foods" is torture—sort of like trimming the guest list for a big party. Even though I have a list of foods that I recommend to clients as my personal all-stars, I hesitate to play favorites. Sure, there are many foods that offer tremendous nutrition, but the six or seven of these foods that are likely to turn into your personal favorites may make someone else hold their nose. (Believe me, bulgur and kefir are amazing, but they turn plenty of people off.) If you won't eat it, it doesn't matter how good it is for you.

So I base my recommendations not just on what's more nutritious but also on what my clients, over the years, have told me they liked the best. All of these foods are also easy to cook with, which is important. Even when we have the best of intentions, there are so many days when we barely have time to use a microwave, let alone soak lentils for 8 hours! I want your pantry and refrigerator to be stocked with simple, healthy, antioxidant-rich tools, not time-consuming projects.

And while the O$_2$ Diet depends on your taking in plenty of fresh produce, the truth is there are days when you just don't have time to go the to supermarket, and all that's left in your crisper is a couple of limp-looking scallions and a few shriveled-up carrots. So this chapter's list includes plenty of foods that can be bought in canned and frozen varieties.

They're not just more convenient—sometimes, they can be cheaper *and* just as nutritious.

You'll recognize lots of these foods from Chapter 2, in which I talked about their specific health benefits. But think of the foods I'm giving you now as nutritional MVPs. You'll notice they don't all contain high amounts of antioxidants. That's because not all great foods do—and they are still vital to eating well. Some grains and protein sources, for example, will have small amounts, while some produce (artichokes, for example) will be off the charts.

Here they are, in alphabetical order. *Mangia!*

Acai berries Juice from these little berries is one of the most nutritious and powerful foods in the world, and can be found in health food and gourmet stores. But I'll be honest—it worries me a little, too. One reason acai has turned into such an overnight sensation is that some companies have claimed it can result in "miraculous" weight loss. Of course that's not true—it's irresponsible to make those claims. But that doesn't mean this juice isn't a tasty, valuable source of antioxidants.

Amaranth Called an "ancient" grain because humans have been raising it for so long, amaranth is high in fiber and nutrient rich. It's loaded with lysine, an essential amino acid the body can't make on its own. (Without it, we develop health problems such as fatigue, anemia, and even kidney stones.)

Avocado This food is actually a fruit, and one that is full of a type of healthy monounsaturated fat you just can't find anywhere else. Avocados may help reduce your risk of developing atherosclerosis and increase your level of that "happy" HDL cholesterol. They have about 20 vitamins, minerals, and beneficial plant compounds, including polyphenols, flavonoids, the antioxidants vitamin E and beta-carotene, as well as plenty of potassium. Plus they're high in fiber . . . and so creamy they taste heavenly. They contain lots of fats, and they taste so good that it's easy to overeat them, especially when you meet up with an amazing guacamole. But you don't have to eat an entire avocado in one sitting—just add fresh lemon or lime juice to avocados after they have been cut, to delay the exposed pulp's darkening, or sprinkle with salt. I chop 1 cup of avocados with 1 cup of tomatoes for a great drip, and I add avocado slices to sandwiches instead of cheese. I even bring half an avocado to the office and eat it with a spoon right at my desk!

Barley High in fiber, this grain actually helps metabolize fats, cholesterol, and carbohydrates. The FDA allows barley products to carry the "may reduce risk of heart disease" label if they contain 0.75 gram of soluble fiber per serving. Some people like barley as a breakfast cereal, either on its own or combined with slow-cooking oats. I love it in soups and as a rice substitute.

Beans These used to get bashed a lot—people either made jokes about gas or called them "poor man's meat." Now we know beans are nutritional superstars, full of flavor, texture, high-fiber complex carbohydrates, low-fat protein, B vitamins, and minerals. The fiber helps to reduce LDL (lousy) cholesterol, aids digestion, and reduces constipation. (And yes, if you eat way more than you're used to, you may get gas.) But fiber also contributes to satiety, that sense of feeling satisfied by what you've just eaten. Satiety protects you from making poor food decisions

Your O$_2$ Breakthrough:
How green is your kitchen?

I like to be as green as possible—not just because it's the right thing to do, but because I care about healthy eating. As we learn more about the most effective environmental practices, though, it's easy to be conflicted. Fishing experts, for example, have pointed out that if everyone in the world ate salmon and other cold-water fish twice a week to protect themselves from heart disease, the oceans couldn't possibly sustain themselves. And those acai berries that are turning up everywhere? Some experts claim we're harming some South Americans by eating so much of this fruit, in effect taking this important food source out of the mouths of very poor (and hungry!) people.[1]

The answers aren't always clear. Ultimately, we all have to make decisions based on our own beliefs, commitment, and budget. (While organic produce has gotten more affordable as it's gotten more popular, it still costs more than conventionally grown food.)

My best advice? Buy as much local produce as you can, and when it fits your budget, choose organic. But pay attention to new thinking. I like to shop at stores like Whole Foods Market and Trader Joe's, which often post signs explaining why they've selected or eliminated certain products.

later. Pair beans with rice or other grains, nuts, cheese, or yogurt; that way you supply the beans' missing amino acids and end up with a dish that is a complete protein. And there are so many yummy varieties to try—I like kidney, black, navy, and pinto beans, chickpeas, and lentils the best.

Beef For meat lovers, there's nothing as mouthwatering as the smell of steak on the grill, and as long as it's a lean cut eaten in a right-size serving (about 4 ounces), it's healthy. In fact, beef is a wonderful source of iron. I like extralean roast beef, top round steak, tenderloin, and fillets. And while it's pricier than conventional beef, I'd urge you to buy grass-fed organic beef, raised without hormones, as often as possible.

Bell peppers Brightly colored bell peppers contain antioxidants and have twice the vitamin C of citrus fruit. (The red, yellow, and orange types also have twice the vitamin C of green peppers.) I like to serve them raw, with hummus or balsamic vinegar, or roast them in the oven, drizzled with olive oil and sea salt. Add them to salads, pasta, or vegetable soup.

Blueberries Their antioxidant power comes from anthocyanins, which may lower LDL cholesterol; pectin, one of the forms of soluble fiber in blueberries, also has cholesterol-lowering properties. (Pectin is helpful in that it adds bulk to stool without stimulating bowel movements.) When buying fresh berries, look for a chalky white color, a "bloom" that signals freshness. Stock up on the frozen berries, too—toss them into smoothies or hot cereal.

Brown rice All rice starts off brown, but traditional processing—milling and polishing—saps much of rice's nutritional value and destroys all its fiber. The processing of brown rice removes only the outermost layer, the hull. Yes, it takes longer to cook brown rice than white rice, but the nutritional benefit is worth it. Try making a batch over the weekend, then storing it, covered tightly, in the fridge, so you can easily use it in meals throughout the week.

Buckwheat Another ancient grain, this one is full of protein and amino acids and can help stabilize blood sugar and reduce hypertension. I like to add buckwheat to salads or use it as a rice substitute.

Bulgur A quick-cooking form of whole wheat, bulgur has been cleaned, parboiled, dried, and ground into particles. It has a yummy, nutty flavor. Often confused with cracked wheat, bulgur differs in that it has been precooked, which means it requires minimal cooking—a must for nights when you're in a rush.

Chicken Chicken is as close to a perfect protein as most of us get. It's affordable, low fat (as long as you stick to white, skinless cuts), easy to prepare, and versatile. There are so many great ways to fix chicken that it never gets dull.

Cinnamon Intensely high in antioxidant value, this spice is thought to control blood sugar in people with diabetes, prevent ulcers, destroy fungal infections, soothe indigestion, ward off urinary tract infections, and fight tooth decay and gum disease. For most of us, just the scent of that gentle spice signals home cooking and comfort food. Sprinkle cinnamon on oatmeal or on fat-free cottage cheese for dessert, use it to make a baked apple, or look for savory recipes—like many Indian dishes—that combine it with other spices.

Citrus fruit Oranges, grapefruit, lemons, tangerines—they're all refreshing and overflowing with vitamin C and other antioxidants. Because they're full of fiber and satisfying to eat—admit it, it's fun to peel an orange or a tangerine at your desk!—they're useful in controlling food cravings.

Corn Whether eaten right off the cob or mixed in black-bean salad, this starchy vegetable isn't just delicious, it's rich in antioxidants. And here's a clear case for buying canned corn: Researchers know that processed corn (because it's cooked at high heat for longer times) is actually higher in antioxidants. Yes, some of its vitamin C is lost in cooking, but the potency of other antioxidants—including ferulic acid, known to help fight cancer—increases dramatically.

Dark chocolate This treat is full of flavonoids, especially catechins, that prevent the buildup of coronary arterial plaque, which is known to contribute to the development of heart disease. (Catechins are also found in tea.) Chocolate boosts your immune system and has anticancer enzymes. But you have to become a label reader, since the way many companies process chocolate, as much as 90 percent of the antioxidants can be lost. Look for products that have at least 60 percent cocoa (70 percent is better) and that list either cocoa beans or cocoa liquor—not some form of sugar!—as the first ingredient. If you can, choose organic chocolate with all natural flavors and ingredients—your taste buds will thank me! And stop torturing yourself with those carob chips—they are no healthier than chocolate.

Eggs This is another dynamite source of protein. I like to buy containers of egg whites to make easy omelets. While the whites are an easy place to get lean protein in your diet, make sure you eat whole eggs sometimes, too. Yes, egg yolks contain all of the egg's fat (about 4.5 grams), but they also contain all of the antioxidants—including vitamins A and E—and more than 90 percent of the vitamins B_6 and B_{12}, as well as important nutrients like calcium, iron, thiamin, and zinc.

Fish Fatty fish, with their essential fatty acids, are a key part of a healthy diet: Salmon, albacore tuna, sardines, and herring can help reduce the risk of developing blood clots, arthritis, cancer, heart disease, and high blood pressure. And while they are lower in fatty acids, don't overlook the great protein found in other fish, including cod, flounder, halibut, sea bass, and tuna. Just be mindful that some fish may be higher in mercury and thus shouldn't be eaten too often.

Flax As with soy, there's some controversy about flaxseed, which is sometimes ground into meal or pressed into oil. I like to recommend flax because it is high in phytoestrogens—especially lignan—thought to protect postmenopausal women from breast cancer. It's also rich in essential fatty acids, including omega-3s, which have well-documented anti-inflammatory properties. They help with blood pressure and may reduce the risk of a heart attack. And they also may help burn fat! Here's the

Your O_2 Moment:
Don't be an orthorectic

Most people have heard of the eating disorders anorexia and bulimia, but experts have discovered a new one—orthorexia, a fixation on the nutritional value of food. As wonderful as it is to choose the best possible foods—those high in antioxidants and other nutrients and those low in fat—it's important to keep it in perspective. Sure, a Golden Delicious apple has fewer antioxidants than a Granny Smith—but both apples are still healthy and, by the way, delicious. Don't let perfect eating be the enemy of the good. Any apple a day keeps the doctor away—no matter what kind it is!

tricky part: Whole flaxseeds usually pass through your body undigested. Buy ground seed or flaxseed oil and add it to salads, yogurt, baked goods, and sauces. My favorite ground flaxseed mix by Spectrum has cranberries, blueberries, and raspberries in it!

Garlic Okay, maybe it's bad for vampires, but it's good for the rest of us. Garlic may protect against stomach and colon cancer, slow the buildup of artery-clogging plaque, prevent the formation of blood clots, help lower blood pressure, reduce the chances of infection, and improve nasal congestion and sinusitis. Simply sauté garlic in olive oil, then add it to soups, dips, and vegetables. Or, to cut down on fat in recipes, sauté it in broth.

Green tea It's tasty, loaded with heart-healthy catechins and other anti-oxidants that aid weight loss—plus it's less caffeinated than many other beverages. I'm not saying you need to replace *all* coffee with this tea, but try to drink at least 2 cups per day, as I recommend in the O₂ Diet.

Ham Pork isn't always fatty, and an extralean ham slice added to sandwiches and salads is a flavorful protein serving.

Honey Yes, the calories in this sweetener can add up quickly, but honey has plenty of nutritional punch and is believed to boost the body's immune system with its antiviral and antibacterial components.

Kale I'm a huge kale fan. If you've never tried it, I urge you to put it at the top of your shopping list. Not only is kale a delicious green, it contains a type of calcium more easily absorbed than those found in other greens: Two cups of cooked kale provides 16 percent of your daily calcium, with only 72 calories. It's also loaded with beta-carotene and vitamin C, has 2.6 grams of fiber, and is a great substitute for spinach. I put it in soups, pasta sauces, stir-fries, and omelets or serve it on its own, sautéed with garlic as a delicious side dish.

Millet Some people flinch when I ask them to try millet. I'll admit, it *is* the main ingredient in bird food. But please don't hold that against it! Millet is delicious, whether eaten as a hot breakfast cereal or served in place of rice or couscous. It contains many of the same goodies that oats do, including heart-protecting manganese, phosphorus, and magnesium—a cup of cooked millet provides 26.4 percent of the daily value for magnesium.

Molasses For the most part, I urge clients to avoid sugar in any form—because most sugars are empty calories. But when you are jonesing for something sweet, try adding a little blackstrap molasses, the darkest kind—a taste you'll probably remember from gingerbread. It's a good source of iron, calcium, copper, manganese, potassium, and magnesium. Try it in a classic recipe: Add a little blackstrap molasses to a pot of beans and bake them.

Nuts and seeds You can't go wrong with a handful of nuts a day—as long as you're grabbing them in calorie-controlled portions. Walnuts, hazelnuts, almonds, pecans, and pistachios all contain healthy fats, which are excellent for your heart. Raw, unsalted nuts and seeds are best and are great tossed into salads, nibbled as a snack, or sprinkled into grain dishes just before serving. I also like to spread nut butters on fiber crackers or apple slices and toss nuts into salads and yogurt. Most of the fat in nuts is monounsaturated, which means it helps manage your cholesterol levels. Nutrition researchers love to quibble about the relative merits of one nut versus another: Walnuts are rich in omega-3 fatty acids, which protect the heart and reduce inflammation, for example. Almonds provide 46 percent of your daily vitamin E requirement. But *all* nuts are good sources of vitamin E, protein, magnesium, calcium, and potassium, and many also contain amino acids that are known to help reduce blood pressure.

But this is why they're my favorites: Nuts provide plenty of satiety. After you snack on a serving—about seven walnut halves, for instance—

Your O$_2$ Injection:
Popeye's secret

That burly sailor man didn't get his strength just from spinach—the secret may have been the can. While many of us have come to look down our noses at canned goods as less nutritious than fresh produce, sometimes canned foods have *more* nutrients: Fresh green beans can lose up to 77 percent of their vitamin C in just 7 days of storage. In some cases, you can radically increase your nutrition by using frozen or canned foods. Canned corn is richer in antioxidants, for example, than fresh or frozen, and canned pumpkin packs 10 times the beta-carotene of fresh.[2]

What are your main triggers?

When it comes to overeating, I'm amazed at what sets different people off. When I do eat poorly, it tends to be because I'm tired (yes, usually because I went too long without a meal!). But everyone is different. From this list, select the two things that are *your* biggest triggers. And promise yourself that for the next month you will pay special attention to protecting yourself from:

- Skipping breakfast
- Eating too fast
- Always finishing a meal with a sweet
- Shopping without a grocery list or when you're hungry
- Not shopping at all, so when you're hungry you have to go out or order in
- Eating in front of the TV or computer
- Picking off your kid's plate
- Snacking on empty calories
- Grazing (eating all day long without listening to your HQ)
- Eating too large a starch or fat serving at a meal
- Going too long between meals

you feel like you ate something nourishing and substantial. And that, of course, protects you from pouncing on the waiter passing around pigs-in-a-blanket at the cocktail party. Hard for you to control your nut nibbling? Many of my clients enjoy measuring nuts into the correct portions and storing them in small zipper-lock bags; that way you are not as tempted to keep nibbling.

Oats They contain about 50 percent more protein than bulgur and twice as much as brown rice, are high in fiber, and help lower cholesterol. Varieties include steel-cut oats, which take longer to cook but have a denser, nuttier texture; rolled oats (instant); and oat bran. Use oats in muffins and pancakes.

Olive oil A monounsaturated fat, this versatile oil may reduce your risk of developing atherosclerosis and breast cancer, and it also contains polyphenols, flavonoids, and the antioxidants vitamin E and beta-carotene. One of the reasons researchers think those who follow a Mediterranean-style diet are so healthy is that they use so much olive oil, and I recommend it instead of saturated fats—honestly, bread dipped in olive oil tastes better than bread with butter! Since it's a fat, it *is* high in calories, so be careful not to use too much. Experiment with herb-infused oils—the extra taste impact can really change a recipe! Go for cold-pressed, extravirgin varieties, which hang on to those valuable heart-healthy polyphenols better than more refined, inexpensive oils. And make sure you know that "extra light" refers to the color of the oil, not the calories.

Onions Along with other alliums, including leeks, scallions, chives, and shallots, onions can help the liver eliminate toxins and carcinogens. And let's be honest—many foods wouldn't be worth eating without the alliums! Some people find chopping onions extremely peaceful, but if the tears drive you crazy, buy prechopped onions to store in the freezer.

Other oils It's a good idea to have other healthy oils on hand, including grapeseed, soybean, walnut, corn, safflower, and sunflower oils. Because they contain essential fatty acids (a type of polyunsaturated fat), they may reduce the risk of developing blood clots, arthritis, cancer, heart disease, and high blood pressure. Just be mindful that most nut oils, while great in salad dressings, lose their nutritional punch at high temperatures. For high-heat cooking, grapeseed oil, with its high "smoke point," is your best bet.

Quinoa This ancient grain, a native to South America but now sold all over, is a rarity among grains—it's a complete protein source, which is another way of saying it has all nine essential amino acids. If I didn't already love quinoa for its protein, I'd adore it because it's also an antioxidant machine—a good source of manganese and copper, two minerals that serve as cofactors for superoxide dismutase enzyme, a key antioxidant the human body manufactures on its own.

Raspberries I love them for their potent antioxidants: One cup provides 6,000 ORAC points and 34 percent of your RDA for vitamin C, plus 8.4 grams of fiber—a third of your daily requirement. They contain pectin, which may help to reduce cholesterol, and they help to stabilize blood sugar. I like them mixed with Greek yogurt and ground flaxseed, and I keep some frozen to toss into smoothies.

Shellfish Mussels, lobster, scallops, shrimp, clams, and oysters are all wonderful, low-calorie protein sources that also contain minerals, including zinc.

Sprouts There are quite a few varieties—alfalfa sprouts, too delicate to cook, and mung bean sprouts, which hold up well in stir-fries. If you've never tried them, look for broccoli sprouts in the market. While all vegetables in the broccoli family (which include cauliflower, kale, and brussels sprouts) have large amounts of the antioxidant sulfurophane, linked to lower cancer risks, broccoli sprouts have the highest amount of all.

Tofu Made from soybeans, this terrific protein source—often called bean curd—is also loaded with isoflavones, which may act as antioxidants to protect your heart and are associated with lower risks of some cancers. It has a cheeselike consistency, but what makes it such a favorite around the world is that it's an amazingly bland food that takes on—beautifully, I might add—the flavors of the foods and spices with which it's cooked.

Tomatoes Whether they're rounding out a salad, perking up a salsa, or topping a pizza, tomatoes are almost universally loved. And they are so good for us—they contain vitamin C, fiber, iron, potassium, and lycopene (a carotenoid that makes tomatoes red), which may help to prevent prostate cancer and heart disease. For maximum lycopene, eat your tomatoes cooked—I like to broil half tomatoes, or sauté cherry or grape tomatoes with garlic and olive oil to serve over fish or chicken. Salsa is great for a snack with carrots and celery sticks.

Turkey It's a shame so many people only think to cook turkey at Thanksgiving—not only is it a great source of lean protein, it's got plenty of B vitamins, iron, zinc, and selenium, a mineral that functions as an antioxidant. As with chicken, most of the fat is in the skin. White meat has less fat than dark meat.

Wild rice Another whole grain option, wild rice has an unusual texture and nutty flavor, and is a good source of manganese and selenium.

Yogurt I know some people are turned off by the consistency, but yogurt is an excellent source of calcium and protein and a good source of riboflavin, phosphorus, and vitamin B_{12}. Yogurt is often easier to digest than milk for people with lactose intolerance. Read labels and avoid fruited yogurt, with added sugar and corn syrup. Instead, select low-fat or fat-free plain yogurt. My favorite: Oikos organic yogurt, which has zero fat.

foods to avoid

Finally—and no, I'm not going to give you a lecture here—there are some foods I want you to swear off for the next 32 days. When you get a craving, remind yourself it's not forever. (But I'm betting that at the end of this month, you will feel so much better that you won't want these foods back in your life anytime soon!)

Bad-for-you baked goods For the next month, avoid all baked goods—and believe me, with the recipes in the O_2 Diet, you won't suffer! Cakes, cookies, muffins, and other sweets are full of calories and often contain the worst kinds of fats—without your even knowing it. I'm not asking you to give up anything for life, but for the next 32 days, we're trying to get rid of as many empty calories as we can to make way for more antioxidants.

Calorie-laden coffees I'm all for a good cup of coffee, but America has gone java-loco for elaborate coffee drinks so loaded with fat and calories that you're practically drinking a milkshake. Some have as many as 1,000 calories!

Sugar-free, fat-free fake-outs There are literally thousands of products that pretend to help people lose weight because they can claim to be fat free or sugar free. The problem is, these foods not only offer little nutrition—okay, does anyone manage to eat those "fat-free" jelly beans with a straight face?—they often aren't even satisfying. So someone will eat four servings of fake dessert and still feel deprived. Fat-free frozen yogurt is a great example: It may not have fat, but it has so many calories from added sugar that it's enough to derail a day of perfect eating. Many sugar-free foods are chock-full of artificial ingredients I can't even pronounce.

Fried-food fiascos Whether it's french fries, fried chicken, or even deep-fried spinach—I swear, this is really served at some restaurants!—

these foods all share one thing in common: They have way too much fat. And often they have way too many empty calories in the form of breading, plus more sodium than anyone needs.

Messy meats Steer clear of high-fat meat choices, including sausage, bacon, ground beef, poultry with skin, and ribs. Not sure? If a cut of beef or lamb looks marbled, that means it's too high in fat.

Nasty nitrates Processed meats—things like hot dogs, salami, and bologna—aren't just high in fat, they're made with nitrates, which have been linked to increased cancer risks. The ones I recommend are nitrate-free.

Sabotaging soft drinks Soft drinks have been linked to obesity and adversely affect bone health. And diet sodas? Sorry, there's no evidence that they're any better for you—there are even studies that suggest that people who drink them are more likely to be obese![3] For the next month, drink water and iced tea. If you are desperate for something fizzy, try a sparkling water.

Scary sweets Avoid all artificial sweeteners just for this month (and actually, I'm hoping you'll feel so good without them that you'll avoid them for life). An important feature of the O₂ Diet is its ability to reawaken your taste buds to the natural sweetness of things like cantaloupe and figs. Plus you'll avoid the frightening list of chemicals that make up these artificial products.

Sneaky sugars Most people are unaware of how much sugar is added into products we don't even think of as all that sweet. Even if you are savvy at spotting safer sugars, like lactose (in milk products) and fructose (found in fruits), be on the lookout for high-fructose corn syrup. Take notice of how much added sugar you eat and the types of food that contain those sugars.

Treacherous trans fats Read labels. If you see the words *hydrogenated* or *partially hydrogenated,* you'll know that food is verboten. Avoid margarine, vegetable shortening, doughnuts, regular peanut butter, and many packaged foods such as cookies, crackers, and chips. There are no beneficial effects from trans fats, but plenty of risks.

8

Your O$_2$ Shopping List

Farmers' markets are my homes away from home. Although it would be nice to eat straight from the sea and the farm all the time, we eventually have to buy food from the grocery store. I like to give my clients specific lists of brands to help them navigate their way through the aisles. The brands listed here are some of my favorites, but there are many more to choose from, and new brands and products pop up every day. Check out www.theO2diet.com for a continually updated grocery list of my favorite food products.

PRODUCE

Fresh Fruit
Fuji apples
Gala apples
Granny Smith apples
Red Delicious apples
Apricots
Avocados (Remember, avocado is really a fat!)
Bananas
Blackberries
Blueberries
Raspberries
Strawberries

Don't forget the superfruits!

While you can easily get 30,000 ORAC points a day from the foods I've already outlined in this book, some people like to dabble in more unusual offerings, including the so-called superfruits. Some of these are from exotic locales; some are American natives but grown in small quantities. If you've got an adventurous spirit, why not track down a few of these at your local health food store for an extra blast of antioxidants, and see if you like them?

Fruit	ORAC per ¼ cup	Health Perks
Goji	14,200	Sometimes called wolfberries, these burnt orange Chinese berries contain zeaxanthin and beta-carotene and may strengthen immune function.
Acai	9,200	Besides its plentiful vitamin C, acai's carotenoids, anthocyanins, and phenolic compounds are thought to be antiviral.
Mangosteen	8,300	Native to Southeast Asia, this fruit contains plenty of xanthones, an antioxidant that may prevent or delay cancer.
Chokeberries	8,100	So sour and acidic that birds won't eat them, these can be blended with other juices to taste great.
Elderberries	5,300	This North American berry has been shown to help lower cholesterol.
Gooseberries	2,100	Along with currants, these tart berries are making a comeback. Juices are good, but also look for them fresh at farmers' markets.
Noni	1,500	This foul-tasting juice from Tahiti has shown some early promise in preventing cancer.

Cantaloupe

Cherries

Figs

Grapefruit

Red grapes

White grapes

Guavas

Honeydew

Kiwifruit

Mangoes

Nectarines

Oranges

Papayas

Passion fruit

Peaches

Pears

Pineapple, extrasweet variety

Plums

Pomegranates

Prunes

Tangerines

Watermelon

Frozen Fruit

Cascadian Farm Organic Blueberries

Cascadian Farm Organic Cherries

Cascadian Farm Organic Strawberries

Sambazon Pure Unsweetened Acai Organic Berry Puree
    Smoothie Packs

Other

Currants

Raisins

Eden Organic Dried Cranberries

Santa Cruz Organic Apple Blackberry Sauce

Santa Cruz Organic Apple Sauce

Shiloh Farms Pitted Bing Cherries

Fresh Vegetables

Corn*

Red potatoes*

Russet potatoes*

Sweet potatoes*

White potatoes*

Butternut squash*

Spaghetti squash*

Alfalfa sprouts

Artichokes

Arugula

Asparagus

Beets

Bok choy

Broccoli

Broccoli rabe

Brussels sprouts

Cabbage

Red cabbage

Carrots

Cauliflower

Celery

Cucumbers

Dandelion greens

Eggplant

Fennel

Garlic

Green beans

Jicama

Kale

Leeks

Boston/Bibb lettuce

Red leaf lettuce

Romaine lettuce

Remember, these are considered starches!

Mushrooms

Red onions

Sweet onions

White onions

Yellow onions

Green bell peppers

Orange bell peppers

Red bell peppers

Yellow bell peppers

Jalapeño chile peppers

Radishes

Scallions

Snow peas

Spinach

Swiss chard

Grape tomatoes

Plum tomatoes

Red tomatoes

Water chestnuts

Watercress

Zucchini

Kombu Seaweed Noodles

Frozen Vegetables

Asparagus

Broccoli

Corn

Peas

Spinach

Cascadian Farm Organic Frozen Mixed Vegetables: Carrots, Corn, and Peas

Columbia River Organics Harvest Trio

Dr. Praeger's Pancakes (Spinach, Broccoli, Sweet Potato)

Seapoint Farms Veggie Blends: Eat Your Greens (My fave!)

Seapoint Farms Veggie Blends: Oriental Blend

GROCERY

Breads

Pumpernickel bread

Whole grain/seven-grain bread

Whole wheat bread

Damascus Bakeries Flax Roll-Ups

French Meadow Bakery Hemp Bread

Nature's Path Organic Pomegran Plus with Oatbran Waffles (frozen)

Rudi's Organic Bakery Whole Grains & Fiber: Wheat & Oat Bread

Thomas' Sahara Mini Whole Wheat Pita Bread

Vermont Bread Company 14 Grains Organic Oat Bread

Vermont Bread Company Oat Bran Oatmeal Bread

Cereals

Steel-cut oats

Arrowhead Mills Instant Oatmeal: Original Plain

Health Valley Organic Fiber 7 Multigrain Flakes

Health Valley Organic Oat Bran Flakes

Kellogg's All-Bran

McCann's Irish Oatbran Hot Cereal

Nature's Path Organic SmartBran with Psyllium & Oat Bran

Quaker Instant Oatmeal

Uncle Sam Instant Oatmeal

Uncle Sam Toasted Whole-Wheat Flakes & Flaxseed Original

Crackers, Chips, and Popcorn

Bearitos Organic No Oil Added Microwave Popcorn

FiberRich Bran Crackers

Garden of Eatin' Microwave Popcorn, no oil added

GG Scandinavian Bran Crispbread

Newman's Own Organics Pop's Corn No Butter/No Salt 94% Fat-Free

Ryvita Rye & Oat Bran Whole Grain Rye Crispbread

Wasa Fiber Rye with Sesame & Oats Crispbread

Grains

Amaranth

Bulgur

Your O$_2$ Breakthrough:
Weird but wonderful

There are a handful of foods that plenty of people might think are weird but that I just love. And they happen to be really nutritious! Why not try:

Black garlic This is conventional garlic that is aged for a month under high heat. It has double the antioxidants of raw garlic, as well as a softer texture and a sweeter taste.

Chia No Chia Pet jokes, please—these seeds are actually a better source of omega-3 fatty acids than flax. Grown in Mexico, and unlike flax, chia seeds don't need to be ground into meal for proper digestion. Sprinkle them in yogurt, cereal, or salads.

Green foods Lots of people think I'm nuts when I recommend things like wheat and barley grasses, which can be bought in powder, tablet, or juice form and offer greater levels of nutrients than green leafy vegetables. I'll be honest: The idea of drinking them makes many of my clients gag. But I don't mind them, and if you can develop a taste for these green foods, they help improve cholesterol levels, blood pressure, and immune response.

Hemp Yes, it's legal! The seeds of this plant, which look like sesame seeds, are another wonderful source of omega-3s and contain plenty of amino acids. You can buy hemp in the form of seeds, oil, or meal.

Kimchi This pickled cabbage delicacy is Korea's national dish. While many people object to the strong flavor, I love it—and it's loaded with antioxidants that include vitamin C and sulforaphane.

Maca Besides its plentiful vitamin C, the powder made from this Peruvian root is packed with carotenoids, anthocyanins, and other phenolic compounds.

Seaweed There are many varieties of edible seaweed, and not only are they rich in minerals but they have lots of antioxidants as well. Fucus (also called bladder wrack) is among the highest, but nori (the most popular) has the most protein, with plenty of calcium, iodine, iron, phosphorus, potassium, manganese, copper, zinc, and vitamins A, B, C, E, and K.

Kamut

Millet

Quinoa

Bob's Red Mill Bulgur

DeBoles Gluten Free Multi Grain Spaghetti Style Pasta Made with Rice, Quinoa, and Amaranth

DeBoles Organic Whole Wheat Angel Hair Made with Jerusalem
   Artichoke Flour
DeBoles Organic Whole Wheat Plus Golden Flax Angel Hair
Eden 100% Buckwheat Soba Noodles
Kretschmer Wheat Germ

Soup
Health Valley Fat-Free Black Bean & Vegetable Soup
Health Valley Fat-Free Chicken Broth
Health Valley Five Bean and Vegetable Soup
Health Valley No-Salt-Added Organic Black Bean Soup
Health Valley Organic 14 Garden Vegetable Fat-Free Soup
Health Valley Organic Potato Leek Soup No Salt Added
Imagine Bistro Organic Cuban Black Bean Bisque
Imagine Natural Creations Light in Sodium Creamy Red Bliss Tomato
   & Roasted Garlic Soup
Imagine Natural Creations Organic Lentil Apple Soup
Imagine Organic Sweet Potato Soup

Other Packaged Foods
Arrowhead Mills Organic Oat Flour
Arrowhead Mills Whole Grain Organic Pastry Flour
Marinated artichoke hearts packed in water (canned or jarred)
Monterey Farms artihearts
Black bean dip
Black beans
Black-eyed peas
Chickpeas
Kidney beans
Lentils
Pinto beans
Split peas
Westbrae beans (My fave!)
Casbah Hummus
Kombu Seaweed Noodles
Libby's 100% Pure Pumpkin

EGGS

The Country Hen Organic Omega-3 Eggs

Horizon Organic Eggs

Land O'Lakes Omega-3 All-Natural Eggs

Organic Valley Organic Large Brown Eggs

Egg Products

Eggology 100% Egg Whites

Gold Circle Farms Cage Free DHA Omega-3 98% Real Eggs
  (liquid egg whites)

Organic Valley Organic Egg Whites

MILK

Hemp Dream Hemp Drink, Original

Hemp Dream Hemp Drink, Vanilla

Oat Dream Oat Drink, Original

Organic Valley Organic Cultured Lowfat Buttermilk

Silk DHA Omega-3 & Calcium, Plain

Silk Light Soymilk, Plain

Silk Soymilk, Plain

Skim Plus Chocolate Milk

Skim Plus Milk

Stonyfield Farm Organic Fat Free Milk

WestSoy Unsweetened Chocolate Soymilk

WestSoy Unsweetened Vanilla Soymilk

YOGURT

Fage Total 0% Greek Yogurt

Oikos Organic Greek Yogurt, Plain

Oikos Organic Greek Yogurt, Vanilla

Silk Plain Soy Yogurt

Stonyfield Farm Light Smoothie

Stonyfield Farm Organic Probiotic Fat-Free Yogurt

True Organic Lactose Free Low Fat Plain Yogurt from Vermont

CHEESE

Cottage cheese (low fat or fat free)

Part-skim mozzarella cheese

Parmesan cheese

Athenos Crumbled Feta with Garlic and Herb

Athenos Crumbled Reduced Fat Feta Cheese

Cabot 50% or 75% Reduced Fat Cheddar

Friendship All Natural Spreadable Low Fat Cottage Cheese 1% Milk
 Fat, Whipped

Lite N' Lively Low-Fat Cottage Cheese

Rachel's Wickedly Delicious Cottage Cheese (Any sweet or savory
 flavor—I love Pear Mangosteen!)

NUTS, NUT BUTTERS, AND SEEDS

Almonds

Brazil nuts

Cashews

Hazelnuts

Macadamia nuts

Peanuts

Pecans

Pine nuts

Pistachios

Sesame seeds

Sunflower seeds

Walnuts

Bob's Red Mill Finely Ground Almond Meal

MaraNatha Natural No Salt Added Creamy & Roasted Almond
 Butter

MaraNatha Natural No Salt Added Creamy & Roasted Cashew
 Butter

MaraNatha Natural No Salt Added Creamy & Roasted Peanut
 Butter

Spectrum Cold Milled Organic Ground Premium Flaxseed

Spectrum Cold Milled Ground Premium Flaxseed with Mixed
 Berries

OILS

Extra virgin olive oil
Colavita 100% Organic Olive Oil
Nutiva Extra-Virgin Coconut Oil
Spectrum Canola Oil
Spectrum Grapeseed Oil
Spectrum Organic Extra Virgin Olive Oil
Spectrum Organic Unfiltered Omega-3 Olive Oil
Spectrum Peanut Oil
Spectrum Safflower Oil
Spectrum Toasted Sesame Oil
Spectrum Walnut Oil

POULTRY

Fresh
Skinless chicken breast
Cornish hen
Fat-free ground turkey
Turkey breast
Applegate Farms Oven Roasted Turkey Breast deli slices

Frozen
Chicken/turkey meatballs
Applegate Farms Organic Turkey Burger
Bell & Evans Grilled Chicken Breasts
Free Bird Grilled Chicken Breast Strips

Other
Applegate Farms Natural Turkey Bacon
Applegate Farms Organic Chicken Hot Dogs
Applegate Farms Organic Turkey Hot Dogs
Han's All Natural Chicken Sausage
SnackMasters Range Grown Natural Turkey Jerky

SEAFOOD

Fresh
Clams
Cod

Flounder

Halibut

King crab

Lobster

Mackerel

Mahimahi

Mussels

Red snapper

Salmon (wild)

Sardines

Scallops

Sea bass

Shrimp

Sole

Tilapia

Tuna

Frozen

Whole catch halibut

Whole catch shrimp in a bag

EcoFish Frozen Coho Alaska Salmon Fillets

EcoFish Frozen Organic Shrimp

St. Dalfour Gourmet On the Go Wild Salmon with Vegetables

Canned or Vacuum Packed

Tuna (canned chunk light in water)

King Oscar Sardines

SnackMasters All Natural Gourmet Ahi Tuna Jerky

SnackMasters All Natural Gourmet Salmon Jerky

Sunkist Tuna Pouch

VitalChoice Albacore Tuna

MEAT

Fresh

Beef sirloin

Beef tenderloin

Flank steak

Ground beef (95% lean)

Extralean ham

Lamb loin

Pork center loin chops

Pork cutlets

Ground pork

Pork tenderloin

Applegate Farms Roast Beef Deli Slices

Applegate Farms Slow Cooked Ham Deli Slices

Great Range Bison Buffalo Steak Medallions

Vegetarian Options

Firm tofu

Tempeh

Dr. Praeger's California Burgers

Gardenburgers

House Foods Tofu Shiritaki Noodles

NaSoya Lite Firm Tofu

Seapoint Farms Edamame Organic Soybeans in Pods

BEVERAGES

Wine

Cabernet

Red

Rosé

White

Tea

Green tea

Celestial Seasonings Black Cherry Berry Herbal Tea

Celestial Seasonings Goji Berry Green Tea

Celestial Seasonings Raspberry Zinger Herbal Tea

Celestial Seasonings Tropical Acai Berry Green Tea

Celestial Seasonings True Blueberry Herbal Tea

The Republic of Tea Daily Green Tea Wild Berry Plum

Traditional Medicinals Organic Roasted Dandelion Root Herbal Tea

Traditional Medicinals Think-O_2 Herbal Dietary Supplement

Juice
Blueberry juice
Cranberry juice
Grape juice
Lemon juice
Lime juice
Pomegranate juice
Prune juice
Tomato juice
Vegetable juice
Hollywood Carrot Juice
Lakewood Organic Heart Healthy Pomegranate with Goji 100%
    Fruit Juice
Lakewood Organic Pomegranate Lemonade
Mountain Sun Grape and Acai
Mountain Sun Pomegranate and Black Cherry
RW Knudsen Family Simply Nutritious Mega Antioxidant Natural
    100% Juice
RW Knudsen Family Simply Nutritious Mega Green Natural 100% Juice
Zico coconut water

Coffee
Whatever you like. I prefer Starbucks Breakfast Blend.

HERBS AND SPICES (I love McCormick and Whole Pantry brands.)
Dried basil leaves
Fresh basil
Black pepper
Cardamom
Chili powder
Chives
Cilantro
Ground cinnamon
Ground cloves
Coriander (cilantro) leaves
Cumin seeds

Curry powder

Fresh dill weed

Garlic powder

Ginger

Ground ginger

Mint leaves

Yellow mustard seed

Nutmeg

Onion powder

Dried oregano leaves

Fresh oregano

Paprika

Parsley

Fresh peppermint

Poppy seeds

Fresh sage

Fresh tarragon

Ground turmeric

CONDIMENTS

Baking powder

Baking soda

Hot cayenne pepper sauce

Canned light coconut milk

Honey

Spicy brown mustard

Pesto

Soy sauce (low sodium)

Turbinado sugar

Oil-packed sun-dried tomatoes

Umeboshi (pickled plums)

Pure vanilla extract

Apple cider vinegar

Brown rice vinegar

Annie's Naturals Organic Pomegranate Vinaigrette

Ba-Tampte White Horseradish
Bragg Organic Healthy Vinaigrette
Buitoni Pesto with Basil
Colavita Marinara Sauce
Cuisine Perel Black Fig Vinegar
Cuisine Perel Blood Orange Vinegar
Cuisine Perel Pomegranate Vinegar
Gourmé Mist Fusions Balsamic Vinegar + Raspberry
Grey Poupon Deli Horseradish Mustard
Grey Poupon Dijon Mustard
Heinz Organic Ketchup
Madhava Agave Nectar
Monari Federzoni Balsamic Vinegar of Modena
Muir Glen Salsa
Real Pickles Organic Red Cabbage
Spectrum Canola Oil Cooking Spray
Spectrum Naturals Organic Golden Balsamic Vinegar
Spectrum Organic Red Wine Vinegar
Spectrum Vegan Caesar Dressing
True Lemon Crystallized Lemon
True Lime Crystallized Lime
True Orange Crystallized Orange

INDULGENCES
Unsweetened dry cocoa powder
Dagoba Organic Chocolate Beaucoup Berries
Emily's Dark Chocolate Covered Blueberries
Green & Black's Hazelnut & Currant Organic Chocolate Bar
Hershey's Chocolate Syrup
NewTree Alpha Thym Dark Chocolate Bar
Sunspire Chocolate-Covered Blueberries
Sweet Riot
TerrAmazon Organic Cacao Powder with Maca

The O₂ Diet Q & A

Q: I don't like math! Do I have to add my ORAC points?

A: I want you to add points for Phase II of the plan because it helps you get in the groove of understanding which foods are highest on the scale. And some people find it helpful to ensure that they keep their ORAC points up each day. For example, you may notice you have only had 25,000 points and are debating between a *conscious indulgence* after dinner that is not as high on the scale and are motivated to go for blueberries instead, since you know that will put you over the 30,000 mark. (Don't forget that you can use your ORAC calculator at www. theO2diet.com to help.) But, if numbers bring back too many bad memories from high school math, you'll like this news: As long as you choose from each food list associated with the building blocks at each meal, you will be eating the right amount of calories *and* foods high in ORAC value.

Q: Should I only eat veggies and other foods from the top of the ORAC list?

A: Eat a variety! All of the foods have many amazing qualities, and some aren't even ORAC-related. Just because a food (a healthy food, that is! I am not talking about French fries!) comes out with a lower ORAC number than another doesn't mean it lacks nutrient value. So, eat a variety from the top and the bottom of lists—I want you to experiment with all kinds of foods that are new to you, too. Also, varying your diet can help you stave off boredom and stay on track. Perhaps if you notice you eat lower ORAC veggies one day—let's say, lots of green salad—aim for the top of the fruit list when choosing a fruit—such as an apple over a pear.

Q: I notice I am supposed to have one portion of fat with my dinner but some of the recipes have more than one fat ingredient?

A: I find that the best way for people to maintain portion control and still eat the right proportion of nutrients is to choose one fat at each meal.That could mean a veggie-loaded salad with lean protein, such as shrimp, and either a serving of avocado OR pecans OR salad dressing. So, when prepping on your own or ordering at a restaurant, you should think this way. However, the O₂ Diet recipes are controlled for you. Even though you may find multiple fats or other ingredients that you thought might have been "off-limits," the recipes are portion-, nutrient- and calorie-controlled. Enjoy!

Q: Are frozen veggies okay?

A: Yes! I wouldn't get my veggies in every single night if it were not for frozen veggies. They are inexpensive and handy and may even have more nutrients than fresh. When veggies are frozen, they are flash frozen and retain many nutrients.

Q: I am a sweetener junkie! Can I still add it to my oatmeal and coffee?

A: *No!* I do not recommend using artificial sweetener. Even though the FDA has approved all sorts of sweeteners, I urge my clients to avoid artificial sweetener—completely! I always tell them to imagine that they've just had a massage at a luxurious spa. What would they feel better drinking in the sauna? A cool glass of water with lemon or a diet soda with its unpronounceable list of chemical additives? While drinking diet sodas and putting artificial sweetener on your yogurt or oatmeal won't add calories, they do expose your body to all kinds of chemicals you don't need. Even worse, these sweeteners just cause you to crave more sweets and distort your natural sense of taste. Once you've gone a few days without them, you will begin to appreciate the natural sweetness of blueberries or even beets! On the naturally sweet side of things, there are plenty of ways to get a sweet fix. You naturally get sugar from foods like fruit, yogurt, and even vegetables. You don't *need* to add ANY to your diet.

Sugar, on the other hand, is hardly a friend, but it is not the evil foe that many make it out to be. The reason sugar gets such a bad rap is that we eat way too much of it, and it is found in way too many foods. Sugar is bad for our teeth and adds pounds to our bodies, often leading to obesity, which we know is related to a plethora of health issues from heart disease to diabetes to cancer. For this reason, I have my clients avoid as much sugar, even natural sugar, as possible. But we all know there are times when you just need a little sweetness. In this case, I recommend less refined sugar such as honey, molasses, agave, or turbinado sugar. You will see honey and turbinado sugar in a few of the O$_2$ Diet recipes. (Turbinado, otherwise known as raw sugar, is made by squeezing fresh cut sugar cane. Since it holds onto some moisture, it has less calories than refined white sugar.) Note that the amount of sugar added to the recipes is very minimal. I have done this math for you, so if you add on your own, *be careful.* Natural or refined sugar calories add up fast! If you do want to go for a noncaloric sweetener because you simply can't give up the sweet taste but don't want the extra calories, then I recommend Stevia. Stevia was recently approved by the FDA and comes from the herb *Stevia rebaudiana.* It has been used in Japan for years!

Q: I don't have a lot of time to prepare healthier snacks or meals. And besides, I don't really like to cook.

A: You don't have to. The convenience craze has swept all across the supermarkets of America, even into the whole-foods aisle. There's no shame in eating many—if not all—of your snacks and meals from foods that are already prepared. I had one client who did just fine using almost nothing but foods that came frozen from the supermarket—vegetables, whole-grain waffles, veggie burgers, even some frozen entrées. (I'm leery of most regular supermarket brands. Calorically they're fine, but they tend to be full of preservatives and sodium.) She didn't even want to be bothered washing fresh fruit, so she used frozen berries! I'm an especially big fan of Cascadian Farms frozen fruits and vegetables, which are organic. For some people, yogurt is just a substitute for a snack they didn't have time to prepare themselves; for others, opening that yogurt counts as cooking. As long as you're keeping focused on the high ORAC foods, keeping your HQ between 4 and 6, getting the right amount of essential nutrients, and losing weight, it's fine.

Q: I can't figure out my HQ.

A: Lots of people struggle with this, especially in the beginning. It's because so many of us are used to eating when we're not hungry. I've had clients confess to me that the only way they can tell they're hungry is when they start snapping at their coworkers, and that the only way they know they're full is when they have to reach down discreetly and unbutton their jeans at the table!

That's why the numbered HQ scale is so helpful (see page 70). *Everyone* can remember what a 1 feels like—that horrible "What-have-I-done, I'm-never-eating-again!" feeling. And most of us can pretty quickly recall a time when we reached 10, allowing ourselves to get so hungry that we felt absolutely frantic. (When that happens to little kids, they often just sit down and howl.)

Now close your eyes and imagine a 5—a completely neutral feeling. You're neither hungry nor full; in fact, at this precise moment, you could care less about food. For the first day, just think in terms of those three scores—1, 5, or 10. But the next time you go to eat something, stop for a second and ask yourself again: Do I feel slightly hungry? Very hungry? Extremely hungry? And after you've finished eating, ask the same questions: Do you feel satisfied? Or like you had a few bites too many?

Your goal—and for some people, it takes a few days—is to recognize when your HQ gets to 6: hungry enough that you feel you should eat something. It's time for a snack or meal. And as you're eating, your goal is to take it slowly enough that you're conscious of your hunger being satisfied. That way, when your HQ hits 4 ("I feel satisfied without a bit of fullness"), you can put down your fork.

Q: I'm traveling. My flight is going to be 6 hours.

A: Travel is tough for many reasons. Besides early check-in and long security lines, airports are notorious for having nothing but overpriced diet disaster zones. Most people spend up to 3 hours without food before they even get on the plane—no wonder there are so many reports of "airport rage"! And once you've fastened your seatbelt, if you get fed at all, chances are your meal will be full of bad fats, sodium, and other chemicals—and taste foul.

As with every other situation, all I can do is urge you to arm yourself with as much healthy food as you think you might need. Don't laugh, but I even suggest that my clients carry snacks aboard in those little insulated lunch bags. (OK, it's about as fashion forward as orthopedic shoes, but it's easy to stash it in your carry-on.) Bring along two or three sets of snacks in case you're delayed. A green apple or portion-controlled bag of pecans. Yogurt can even be left out for a couple of hours, but you must buy that once you get through security, along with water. And don't forget lemon; True Lemon makes great little lemon packets that you can easily throw in that little plastic baggie when you run your cosmetics through security. And remember, try to eat a "real" meal as close to departure as possible to save the snacks you brought along in case you get stuck at your terminal.

I even suggest that clients fill their luggage with plenty of nonperishable snack foods: Try buffalo jerky, trail mix (18 pistachios and 2 chopped dried apricots), oatmeal packets, tuna packets, green tea bags. It will help keep you closer to your routine while traveling.

Q: I'm starting to plateau.

A: Most people will lose between 8 and 10 pounds in the first month of the O_2 Diet, more if they've got more weight to lose and if they haven't been on other diets recently. (That's because chronic dieting meddles with people's metabolism, and it can take a few weeks of following a healthy diet for it to get back to normal.) But it can be very frustrating, especially as you get closer and closer to your goal weight, to have weight loss slow to less than a pound a week.

The only thing I can do is urge you to remember that weight loss is a long-term process. This is not something you'll work on for a month and then forget all about. The O_2 Diet is about long-term changes not only to how you look and what you weigh on the scale but also to how you feel. You probably didn't gain the weight in a month-long period, so it's not realistic to expect to lose it that quickly. And—remember as tedious as it is—there's plenty of evidence that the more slowly you shed those extra pounds, the more likely they are to stay gone. Be patient and consistent!

Q: I'm not losing weight.

A: Not losing weight at all is different from losing weight too slowly. If you've been on the O_2 Diet for a week and haven't lost any weight, it's time to reassess. First, look back at your food journals, retracing your steps each day. One client, for example, kept forgetting to record the cappuccinos she ordered twice a day at work. Even thought they were made with skim milk, they added 200 invisible calories per day—enough to prevent her from losing weight.

Next, double-check the portions of food you're eating. Even if you've been eating nothing but big salads, ask yourself if they've gotten a little *too* big. Too much chicken thrown in? Overdoing the dressing? Even overeating the good stuff can interfere with weight loss.

Q: By the way, I hate using my food journal. Can I stop?

A: Sorry, but I would like you to keep on food journaling even if you stop adding up ORAC points. When people record what they eat, they often find they've been drastically underestimating their intake, according to a study published in the *New England Journal of Medicine*. And I know, it is embarrassing to write down all the weird and inexplicable ways we cheat. (Believe me, there is nothing I haven't seen on these food diaries, from "half a container of Duncan Hines frosting with celery" to "nutrition bars dipped in peanut butter!")

Need more evidence? A study done at the University of Pennsylvania School of Medicine found that dieters who kept food journals lost more weight in the weeks in which they recorded their food the most accurately and less in weeks where they were sloppier. I tell my clients daily: Not only can I help you more, but you will help yourself more if you write it down. You get the point: No matter what you eat, *write it down*.

Q: What if I overeat? Do I skip eating the next day?

A: Never skip a meal or force yourself to go hungry—that kind of penance-and-reward system just doesn't work.

Remember the O_2 Diet is about empowering yourself! Not beating yourself up! Every time you "fall off the wagon," whether it's because you ate too much of a recommended food or a food that's not recommended at all, just record it and calmly move on. Every snack, every meal is a new page, a totally clean slate. And nobody is perfect.

This is a good time to revisit the black-and-white thinking that sabotages so many diets. It's so easy for us to say, "I blew it—not only did I have pizza instead of the salad, I had three pieces. I might as well keep eating like a maniac all weekend and start over on Monday."

There's no reason to punish yourself like that. I know it's corny, but I sometimes ask clients to visualize that way babies learn to walk. When they fall down, do they lie there and kick and scream and decide they won't try again until Monday morning, or until January 1? Of course not. They fuss a little, then pull themselves back up and try again. The O$_2$ Diet involves the same process. This isn't the way you're used to eating, so you may make mistakes, probably more than a few times. That's okay.

Q: Since you say I can eat as many veggies as I want, can I have a salad with dinner every night?

A: Yes! As long as you are not adding extra fat servings such as toppings like cheese and/or salad dressing. Not only can you have the salad, but I want you to add a salad! Having a salad to start and a veggie with your meal means you will be packing in extra antioxidants. Also, veggies have fiber, which you know by now helps to keep you full without adding lots of extra calories. For a change, simply make or order a side of any veggie you like as a substitute for a salad. Either way, up the veggies!

For more O$_2$ Diet Q & A, go to www.theO2diet.com.

More O$_2$ Questions and Answers!

For the paperback edition of *The O$_2$ Diet,* I put together some of the most common questions I received from readers. Here they are. I hope they help!

Q: During the cleanse, can I still drink my 2 cups of black coffee in the morning?

A: Yes! One or 2 cups of black coffee is fine. If coffee keeps you up at night or makes you feel jittery, I would stay away from it. But if you are only drinking 1 or 2 cups in the morning and have no side effects, go for it, as long as you don't add sweetener (artificial or real) and milk or creamer to it. After the cleanse, you can certainly add skim or light soy milk. And don't forget, I still want you to get in your 2 cups of green tea each day.

Q: Is it acceptable to use jarred or canned foods? I know it's better to buy fresh or frozen foods, but it can get very expensive.

A: Canned is okay! Canned foods sometimes contain even more antioxidants than fresh or frozen. (For example, canned corn is richer in antioxidants than fresh or frozen, and canned pumpkin packs 10 times the beta-carotene of fresh.) When you do go for canned foods, choose the option that has the least amount of sodium and is packed in water. One negative to canned foods is that they may contain the chemical BPA. However, you can look for BPA-free canned items, so choose canned goods marked "BPA-free" whenever possible. Whether you choose fresh, canned, or frozen, be sure to get your fruits and veggies in any way you can.

Q: What if I don't like one of the vegetables used in your recipes? For instance, I absolutely cannot stomach artichokes.

A: Swap it out for a veggie you love. Just refer to your ORAC veggie list and try to find one you like that is high in ORAC points and that you will enjoy the taste of in place of the one you don't like. Enjoy your food! There is no forcing yourself to eat something you do not like on the O_2 diet!

Q: Is there a way to follow the O_2 diet while also being vegetarian or vegan? I'm especially concerned about what I can eat in place of meat, poultry, fish, eggs, etc. Help!

A: Absolutely! A vegetarian lifestyle can be a very healthy one when you make conscious food choices. Vegetarians suffer significantly lower mortality from heart disease than health-conscious nonvegetarians do. Research shows that mortality from ischemic heart disease is 57 percent lower in vegetarians than in the general population. Following the O_2 diet as a vegetarian is a very good way to ensure that you are meeting all of your dietary needs. Any lean vegan protein will do as a substitute for meat, poultry, fish, and eggs. For example, instead of eggs at breakfast, use firm tofu.

Q: Can I follow the O_2 diet while on a gluten-free diet?

A: Absolutely! In fact, the majority of the foods on the O_2 diet are gluten-free. When choosing a starch, simply choose one that is right for you, such as millet, quinoa, or brown rice. In any recipe that calls for a food that is not gluten-free, you can simply swap that ingredient for the same portion of an alternate starch. I think you will be happy to find that you'll need to make very few substitutions.

Q: I want to follow this plan but I have food allergies, specifically to dairy, soy, and eggs. How can I properly substitute foods and still remain on the plan?

A: No problem! In place of dairy, substitute unsweetened almond, hemp, or rice milk. In place of soy products and eggs in recipes, substitute another lean protein. For example, on the cleanse, try having three slices of turkey for breakfast instead of eggs.

More O_2 Questions and Answers!

Q: Is the O_2 diet appropriate for someone with diabetes? I have been diagnosed with type 2 diabetes and have been controlling my blood sugar through diet, but I need to lose some weight, as well.

A: The O_2 diet is a low-glycemic diet, so it's definitely appropriate for someone with diabetes. It is very low in refined sugars, low in sugar in general, and it also provides nutrients in the proper proportions for a diabetic. In addition, on the O_2 diet you eat consistently throughout the day, which helps you maintain proper blood sugar levels.

Q: I have diverticulosis and cannot eat any nuts or any fruits containing seeds, which means most berries are off-limits! Is it possible to substitute other foods and still follow your plan?

A: Absolutely! You can swap out the nuts for any other healthy fat, such as avocado, and the berries can be replaced with any other high-ORAC fruit, such as mango. You will still reap the benefits with these substitutions.

Q: Are there specific modifications or adjustments I should make for pregnancy?

A: Congratulations! You can absolutely follow the plan while you're pregnant. Add in one extra starch serving and one additional fruit or milk/yogurt serving. And of course, listen to your body. If you are truly hungry, adjust. If you have a true craving, try to satisfy it with a *conscious indulgence.*

Q: Are there any supplements you recommend taking? If so, which do you recommend?

A: Food always comes first, and supplements should never take the place of "real" food. However, I do recommend supplements as "insurance." My recommendations vary for each person, but in general I recommend a multivitamin and an omega-3 supplement. Then, depending on your unique needs, I sometimes recommend a calcium plus vitamin D supplement, a probiotic, and other supplements as necessary.

Q: Do I have to begin with the 4-day cleanse in order to progress through the O$_2$ diet? I am not looking to lose any weight, but I really want to increase the amount of antioxidants I eat to be healthier in general.

A: The O$_2$ diet is perfect for someone like you! It is truly a healthy lifestyle that will help you lose weight *if* you are overweight but will also help improve general health. What you should do if you do not want to lose weight is skip the 4-day cleanse and even Phase 1, if you like; go straight to weeks 3 and 4 of the diet. I get so excited when people simply want to be *healthy!*

Q: Do I have to eat each meal and snack the way they're laid out in your plan? What if I'm not hungry? Am I allowed to have one of my snacks after dinner, instead?

A: As long as you are getting the correct number of servings from each food group, listening to your body, and eating consistently throughout the day, it's perfectly fine to base your meals and snacks around your schedule and what works best for you.

Q: How many calories are provided on the O$_2$ diet? I have followed 1,200-calorie plans in the past, and they've helped me lose weight. I'm struggling to lose these last 10 pounds and want to make sure I'm within an appropriate calorie range to help me push past this plateau.

A: This plan provides 1,200 to 1,500, depending upon the phase you are in, the amount of protein you consume, and whether or not you have had a *conscious indulgence* that day.

Q: Am I allowed to chew gum?

A: You can't have gum with sugar in it because of the extra calories and tooth decay. I'm also not a fan of sugar-free gum, as gum chewing in general can cause bloat, and for some people, chewing gum can trigger appetite. For others, of course, it may help curb a craving. It varies by individual, but I would suggest avoiding gum if possible. Try to satisfy your oral fixation by sipping tea or crunching on celery.

Q: I am very social and go out a lot for work. Can I drink alcohol?

A: Alcohol is what I consider a *conscious indulgence*. During Phase III you add in one *conscious indulgence*, and then during O$_2$ for life, you add in another. Alcohol in moderation has many health benefits. If you enjoy alcohol, make it your *conscious indulgence* and be aware of how you feel when you drink. Does it make you want to eat more? Be aware of that, and choose lower-calorie cocktails. No fruity drinks!

Q: I have tried every diet ever created! I want to do it right this time, but I've heard that once you have dieted it is harder to lose weight the next time. Is this true?

A: Having dieted in the past can be your best advantage or your weakest link. It is true that the more you diet the more damage you can do to your metabolism. However, knowing what has worked and what hasn't worked for you in the past can be a huge asset this time around. Go for it! On the O$_2$ diet, you'll make changes that you can stick with for life.

Q: I love water with lemon but want to add a no-calorie sweetener. Is that okay?

A: No! Water is pure goodness! Lemon is pure vitamin C! Don't take away from doing good for your body by adding an artificial sweetener. These chemicals will do you no good and may even cause harm, including setting you up for greater cravings later in the day. If you are using sweetener now, cut it in half. Then challenge yourself to go sweetener-free for 3 days. I bet you won't want to go back!

Breakfast
PHASE II

Cocoa-Nut Smoothie

1 cup fat-free plain yogurt

$\frac{1}{2}$ small banana, cut into 1" pieces

$\frac{1}{4}$ cup Zico Coconut Water

2 teaspoons smooth almond butter

2 teaspoons unsweetened cocoa powder

2 teaspoons vanilla extract

1 teaspoon flaxseed oil

1. Place the yogurt, banana, coconut water, almond butter, cocoa, vanilla, and oil in a blender. Puree about 10 seconds or until smooth.
2. Serve sprinkled with additional cocoa powder, if desired.

Makes 1 serving

ORAC Value: 3,980

Genesis Today Purple Perfection Smoothie

(adapted from Genesis Today)

2 ounces Genesis Today Acai Berry Juice

2 ounces Genesis Today Resveratrol Juice

$\frac{1}{2}$ small banana, cut into 1" pieces

$\frac{3}{4}$ cup plain fat-free yogurt

2 teaspoons almond butter

5 ice cubes

1. Place the acai juice, resveratrol juice, banana, yogurt, almond butter, and ice cubes in a blender. Pulse until smooth and well combined.

Makes 1 serving

ORAC Value: 4,306

Barley Breakfast Salad

3 tablespoons fat-free ricotta cheese

$\frac{1}{4}$ teaspoon pure maple syrup or honey

$\frac{1}{4}$ teaspoon ground cinnamon, divided

$\frac{1}{3}$ cup cooked quick-cooking pearl barley

1 tablespoon chopped pecans

1 teaspoon dried cranberries

1 medium orange, sectioned and cut into $\frac{3}{4}$" pieces

$\frac{1}{2}$ teaspoon orange zest

1. Combine the ricotta, maple syrup or honey, and $\frac{1}{8}$ teaspoon of the cinnamon in a small bowl. Set aside.
2. Combine the barley, pecans, cranberries, orange, zest, and the remaining $\frac{1}{8}$ teaspoon of cinnamon in a serving bowl. Top with the ricotta mixture. Sprinkle with additional cinnamon, if desired.

Makes 1 serving

ORAC Value: 10,225

Huevos Rancheros

$\frac{1}{2}$ teaspoon olive or canola oil

$\frac{1}{4}$ cup canned black beans, rinsed and drained

2 tablespoons salsa, divided

$\frac{1}{4}$ teaspoon ground cumin

$\frac{1}{8}$ teaspoon chili powder

1 tablespoon chopped cilantro, divided

1 large omega-3-enriched egg

Pinch salt and freshly ground black pepper

1 small (5") corn tortilla

1 tablespoon shredded Mexican blend cheese

Hot sauce (optional)

1. Heat the oil in a small nonstick skillet over medium heat. Use a paper towel to spread the oil evenly over the surface.
2. Use a fork to mash the beans with 1 tablespoon of the salsa. Add the cumin, chili powder, and 2 teaspoons of the cilantro. Set aside.
3. Add the egg to the skillet and season with salt and pepper. Cook for 1 to 2 minutes, or until the white is completely cooked through.
4. Place the tortilla between two damp paper towels and heat it in the microwave for 30 seconds or until warmed through.
5. Lay the tortilla flat on a serving plate and spread the bean mixture evenly on top, leaving $\frac{1}{4}$" around the edge. Use a spatula to loosen and transfer the egg to the top of the bean mixture.
6. Sprinkle the egg with the cheese, then top with the remaining 1 tablespoon of salsa and 1 teaspoon of cilantro and serve immediately. Drizzle with hot sauce, if desired.
7. Serve with pineapple chunks on the side.

Makes 1 serving

ORAC Value: 5,915

Lunch

Avocado and Cucumber Nori Rolls with Cashew-Carrot Dipping Sauce

SAUCE

$1/2$ medium carrot, cut into 1" pieces

2 teaspoons chopped cashews

$1/2$ teaspoon minced ginger

1 tablespoon rice wine vinegar

1 tablespoon water

$1/2$ teaspoon sesame oil

Pinch sea salt

NORI ROLLS

$1/2$ medium carrot

$1/2$ medium cucumber

2 sheets roasted seaweed

$2^1/2$ teaspoons plain hummus

$1/4$ avocado, cut lengthwise into 4 pieces, each about $1/4$" thick

1. *To make the sauce:* Combine the carrot, cashews, ginger, vinegar, water, oil, and salt in a blender or food processor fitted with a metal blade. Puree for 15 seconds, or until the carrots are finely grated, scraping down the sides halfway through. Set aside.

2. *To make the nori rolls:* Peel the carrot lengthwise, removing a thin layer of the skin. Place the cut side down and repeat on all remaining sides. Cut it in half lengthwise, then cut each half into 2 pieces, each about $1/4$" thick. Peel the cucumber lengthwise, removing a thin layer of the skin from all sides. Cut it lengthwise into 4 pieces, then stack 2 pieces flat on top of each other and cut them into 4 thin strips. Repeat with the remaining 2 pieces. Cut a sheet of plastic wrap slightly larger than a sheet of seaweed. Lay one seaweed sheet flat on the plastic wrap vertically. Place 4 pieces of cucumber flush with the bottom edge of the sheet, and place 4 more pieces next to them. Then place 1 piece of carrot next to the cucumbers on each side. Add $1/2$ teaspoon of hummus next to each carrot, and finally place 1 piece of avocado next to the hummus on each side. (Cut the ends of the veggies if necessary, so that they won't poke out of the roll.)

3. Repeat with the second sheet of seaweed and the remaining cucumbers, carrots, hummus, and avocado.
4. Use the plastic wrap to carefully lift the seaweed end that's closest to you (the filling should come right to the edge) and tightly roll it away from yourself, making sure the contents remain inside the roll at the ends. Dot the edge with $\frac{1}{4}$ teaspoon of the remaining hummus to seal, and turn the roll seam-side down. Repeat with remaining roll.
5. Cut each roll into 4 pieces. Serve with the dipping sauce and edamame on the side.

Makes 1 serving

ORAC Value: 7,381

Green Goddess Edamame Salad & Dressing

DRESSING

2 tablespoons fat-free plain yogurt

1 tablespoon finely chopped, shelled, raw pistachios

1 tablespoon steeped green tea, cooled to room temperature

1 tablespoon thinly sliced green onion

1 teaspoon finely chopped parsley

1 teaspoon red wine vinegar

$\frac{1}{2}$ teaspoon minced garlic

Salt and freshly ground black pepper

SALAD

$\frac{3}{4}$ cup frozen, shelled edamame

$\frac{1}{2}$ cup celery, thinly sliced

$\frac{1}{3}$ cup chopped marinated artichoke hearts

$\frac{1}{4}$ cup thinly sliced radishes

1. *To make the dressing:* Place the yogurt, pistachios, tea, onion, parsley, vinegar, and garlic in a small bowl. Season to taste with salt and pepper. Set aside.
2. *To make the salad:* Defrost the edamame in the microwave according to the package directions. Let it cool to room temperature.
3. Toss the edamame, celery, artichoke hearts, and radishes with the dressing and serve.

Makes 1 serving

ORAC Value: 15,423

Sausage & Peppers Pita

1 teaspoon olive oil

$\frac{1}{2}$ small green or red bell pepper, cut into $\frac{1}{4}$"-thick strips (about 6 strips)

$\frac{1}{4}$ cup thinly sliced red onion

$\frac{1}{3}$ cup thinly sliced button mushrooms

1 Applegate Farms Organic Sweet Italian Chicken and Turkey Sausage

1 teaspoon Dijon mustard

1 tablespoon plain hummus

1 oat bran pita (6")

Freshly ground black pepper

1. Heat the oil in a medium nonstick skillet or grill pan over medium-high heat. Add the peppers and onions in a single layer. Cover and cook for 5 minutes.
2. Toss the peppers and onions and add the mushrooms to the skillet. Place the sausage in with the vegetables and cook for 8 to 10 minutes, turning occasionally, until the vegetables are softened and the sausage is heated through.
3. Combine the mustard and hummus in a small bowl. Top the pita with the sausage, mustard mixture, and vegetables. Season with pepper to taste.

Makes 1 serving

ORAC Value: 2,110

Dinner

Quinoa Stuffed Pepper

1 medium red or green bell pepper

$\frac{1}{3}$ cup cooked quinoa

$\frac{1}{3}$ cup chopped tomatoes

$\frac{1}{3}$ cup grated zucchini

1 tablespoon minced basil or parsley

2 tablespoons grated Parmesan or Romano cheese, divided

1 tablespoon pine nuts, divided

1 teaspoon lemon juice

1 teaspoon olive oil

$\frac{1}{2}$ teaspoon minced garlic

Salt and freshly ground black pepper

1. Preheat the oven to 375°F.
2. Cut the top off of the bell pepper and remove the seeds and ribs, leaving the remaining pepper intact. Trim the bottom slightly, if necessary, so it will stand up straight.
3. Combine the quinoa, tomatoes, zucchini, basil or parsley, 1 tablespoon of the cheese, 2 teaspoons of the pine nuts, lemon juice, oil, and garlic in a medium bowl. Season with salt and black pepper to taste.
4. Place the bell pepper in a baking dish and add enough water to come halfway up the sides of the dish.
5. Cover with foil and bake for 30 minutes. Top the pepper with the remaining 1 tablespoon of cheese and 1 teaspoon of pine nuts and bake, uncovered, for 15 more minutes or until the cheese is melted and the nuts are golden.

Makes 1 serving

ORAC Value: 1,975

Green Tea–Marinated Cod over Lentil-Currant Salad

2 tablespoons freshly squeezed lemon juice

1 tablespoon fig vinegar

$\frac{1}{4}$ cup steeped green tea, cooled to room temperature

$\frac{1}{2}$ teaspoon minced ginger

$\frac{1}{2}$ teaspoon honey

$\frac{1}{2}$ teaspoon olive oil

$\frac{1}{2}$ teaspoon Dijon mustard

3 tablespoons finely chopped shallots

Salt and freshly ground black pepper

4-ounce cod fillet (about $\frac{3}{4}$" thick), cut into 4 uniform cubes

$\frac{1}{3}$ cup cooked or canned lentils, rinsed and drained

$1\frac{1}{2}$ cups baby spinach

2 teaspoons dried currants

1 bamboo skewer, 8" long

1. Combine the lemon juice, vinegar, tea, ginger, honey, oil, mustard, and 2 tablespoons of the shallots in a medium bowl. Season with salt and pepper to taste.
2. Reserve 2 tablespoons of the marinade to use as a dressing, and set aside.
3. Place the fish in the bowl with the remaining marinade. Cover and refrigerate for 15 minutes.
4. While the fish marinates, soak the bamboo skewer in water.
5. Lightly mist a grill pan or medium nonstick skillet with canola oil cooking spray and place it over medium heat.
6. Thread the fish onto the skewer. Cook for 5 minutes or until the fish is opaque, using a spatula to carefully flip the skewer halfway through.
7. Toss the lentils, spinach, currants, and the remaining 1 tablespoon of shallots with 1 tablespoon of the dressing. Place the skewer on top of the salad and drizzle the remaining dressing on top of the fish. Serve immediately.

Makes 1 serving

ORAC Value: 10,837

"Better" Bison Taco Salad with Spicy Chipotle Dressing

2 tablespoons fat-free plain yogurt

1 teaspoon freshly squeezed lime juice

1 canned chipotle chile pepper in adobo (or $\frac{1}{4}$ teaspoon ground chipotle chile pepper)

$1\frac{1}{2}$ teaspoons olive oil, divided

$\frac{1}{4} + \frac{1}{8}$ teaspoon ground cumin

$\frac{1}{4}$ teaspoon paprika

4-ounce bison sirloin steak

$\frac{1}{8}$ teaspoon ground chili powder

$\frac{1}{8}$ teaspoon sea salt

Freshly ground black pepper

$1\frac{1}{2}$ cups chopped romaine lettuce

$\frac{1}{3}$ cup canned kidney beans, rinsed and drained

$\frac{1}{4}$ cup chopped red bell pepper or tomatoes

1 tablespoon Mexican blend or shredded Monterey Jack cheese

2 tablespoons chopped red onion

1. *To make the dressing:* Puree the yogurt, lime juice, chipotle chile pepper, 1 teaspoon of the oil, $\frac{1}{4}$ teaspoon of the cumin, and $\frac{1}{8}$ teaspoon of the paprika in a blender or food processor fitted with a metal blade until smooth. Set aside.
2. *To make the taco salad:* Preheat a medium nonstick skillet or grill pan over medium heat. Rub the steak with the chili powder, sea salt, the remaining $\frac{1}{8}$ teaspoon of cumin, and the remaining $\frac{1}{8}$ teaspoon of paprika. Drizzle with the remaining $\frac{1}{2}$ teaspoon of olive oil to coat both sides, and season with black pepper to taste.
3. Toss the lettuce, beans, bell pepper or tomato, cheese, and red onion in a medium bowl.
4. Cook the steak for about 2 minutes per side for medium. Remove from the heat and let stand for 5 minutes before slicing into $\frac{1}{4}$"-thick pieces.
5. Toss the salad with the prepared dressing and place the steak on top. Serve immediately.

Makes 1 serving

ORAC Value: 8,145

Your O₂ Life Journal

Name: _____

Date:		ORAC Total
Sleep:		
Exercise:		
Pampering:		
Fluid:	Green tea __ x 3,000 = _____ H₂O with lemon __ x 400 = _____	
Breakfast: Time: HQ:		
Snack: Time: HQ:		
Lunch: Time: HQ:		
Snack: Time: HQ:		
Dinner: Time: HQ:		
ORAC TOTAL:		

Your O₂ Life Journal

Name: _____

Date:		ORAC Total
Sleep:		
Exercise:		
Pampering:		
Fluid:	Green tea __ x 3,000 = _____ H₂O with lemon __ x 400 = _____	
Breakfast: Time: HQ:		
Snack: Time: HQ:		
Lunch: Time: HQ:		
Snack: Time: HQ:		
Dinner: Time: HQ:		
ORAC TOTAL:		

Your O₂ Life Journal

Name: _____

Date:		ORAC Total
Sleep:		
Exercise:		
Pampering:		
Fluid:	Green tea __ x 3,000 = _____ H₂O with lemon __ x 400 = _____	
Breakfast: Time: HQ:		
Snack: Time: HQ:		
Lunch: Time: HQ:		
Snack: Time: HQ:		
Dinner: Time: HQ:		
ORAC TOTAL:		

Your O₂ Life Journal

Name: _____

Date:		ORAC Total
Sleep:		
Exercise:		
Pampering:		
Fluid:	Green tea __ x 3,000 = _____ H_2O with lemon __ x 400 = _____	
Breakfast: Time: HQ:		
Snack: Time: HQ:		
Lunch: Time: HQ:		
Snack: Time: HQ:		
Dinner: Time: HQ:		
ORAC TOTAL:		

Your O₂ Meal Planner

Use this worksheet to plan your meals ahead for the week. Plan your *conscious indulgences*, which meals you're going to cook, and which meals you'll eat out.

	Monday	Tuesday	Wednesday	
Date	_ / _ / _	_ / _ / _	_ / _ / _	
Breakfast				
Snack				
Lunch				
Snack				
Dinner				

	Thursday	Friday	Saturday	Sunday
	_ / _ / _	_ / _ / _	_ / _ / _	_ / _ / _

Your O$_2$ Shopping List

Copy this page and fill it in before going to the grocery store. This will help you make sure you don't forget any of the O$_2$ foods you want to include in your meals for the week ahead. Planning is essential!

Your O$_2$ Shopping List	Date: _____
Fruit	Vegetables
Starches	Lean Proteins
Milk, Yogurt, and Soy	Fats
Beverages	Herbs, Spices, and Condiments

Glossary

Because there is so much ongoing research in the world of nutrition and antioxidants, defining basic terms—let alone clarifying the evidence about what they may be able to do for your health—can be confusing. I've collected these definitions from some of the most reliable, acceptable sources, relying heavily on Medline, maintained by the US National Institutes of Health; the International Food Information Council Foundation; the Linus Pauling Institute at Oregon State University; and the *Health & Nutrition Newsletter* published by the Friedman School of Nutrition Science and Policy at Tufts University; as well as the American Heart Association, the American Cancer Society, the National Cancer Institute, the American Institute for Cancer Research, the US Agricultural Research Service, and the Alzheimer's Association.

I also like to use Web sites run by the Mayo Clinic, the Cleveland Clinic, and WebMD, because they cover the connection between nutrition research and health in an accurate, user-friendly way.

If you'd like to learn more, all these resources are available to the public, at no cost. Go to www.theO2diet.com and click on Resources for links to these and other sources.

allium, alliinase Garlic is a particularly rich source of these organosulfur compounds, which are currently under investigation for their potential to prevent and treat disease. Crushing or chopping garlic releases an enzyme called alliinase that catalyzes the formation of allicin. Allicin rapidly breaks down to form a variety of organosulfur compounds.

alpha-lipoic acid See lipoic acid.

amino acids The basic building blocks of proteins, some amino acids are classified as essential, which means we need them in our diet. These include histidine, isoleucine, leucine, lysine, methionine, phenylalanine, threonine, tryptophan, valine, and possibly arginine. Nonessential amino acids are synthesized by the body and include alanine, asparagine, aspartic acid, glutamic acid, glutamine, glycine, proline, and serine.

anthocyanins This group of antioxidants is a subclass of flavonoids, which provide the health benefits of neutralizing free radicals and possibly reducing the risk of cancer. Anthocyanins are found in red, blue, and purple berries; red and purple grapes; and red wine. They include cyanidin, delphinidin, malvidin, pelargonidin, peonidin, and petunidin.

antioxidants Substances that protect your cells against the effects of free radicals. Free radicals are molecules produced when your body breaks down food or by environmental exposures such as tobacco smoke and radiation, which damage cells and contribute to aging, heart disease, cancer, and other diseases. Antioxidants protect key cell components by neutralizing the damaging effects of free radicals.

ascorbic acid Also known as vitamin C, this water-soluble vitamin is essential for the development and maintenance of connective tissue and to speed the production of new cells in wound healing. It is also an antioxidant that keeps free radicals from hooking up with other molecules to form damaging compounds that might attack tissue. Vitamin C protects the immune system, helps fight off infections, reduces the severity of allergic reactions, and plays a role in the synthesis of hormones and other body chemicals. Food sources include green bell peppers, broccoli, citrus fruits, tomatoes, and strawberries.

atherosclerosis A condition that exists when too much cholesterol builds up in the blood and accumulates in the walls of the blood vessels.

beta-carotene A derivative of the antioxidant vitamin A, this compound is found in many foods that are orange in color, including sweet potatoes, carrots, cantaloupe, squash, apricots, pumpkin, and mangos. Some green leafy vegetables (including collard greens, spinach, and kale) are also rich in beta-carotene.

body mass index (BMI) A method of determining overweight and obesity. BMI is a calculation that divides a person's weight in pounds by height in inches, squared. Search the term "BMI" for many calculators on the Internet, or use this formula: BMI = [lbs/in²] x 703. The general guideline currently iterated by the Centers for Disease Control and Prevention is that individuals with a BMI of 25 to 29.9 are considered overweight and those with a BMI of 30 or greater are considered obese.

caffeic acid A type of phenol found in various fruits (including citrus) and vegetables, caffeic acid has antioxidant-like activities and may reduce the risk of degenerative diseases, heart disease, and eye disease.

caffeine A naturally occurring substance found in the leaves, seeds, or fruits of more than 63 plant species worldwide, caffeine is part of a group of compounds known as methylxanthines. The most commonly known sources of caffeine are coffee and cocoa beans, kola nuts, and tea leaves. Caffeine is a pharmacologically active substance and, depending on the dose, can be a mild central nervous system stimulant. Caffeine does not accumulate in the body over the course of time and is normally excreted within several hours of consumption. Coffee is the primary source of antioxidants in the United States.

calcium A mineral that builds and strengthens bones, calcium helps in muscle contraction and heartbeat and assists with nerve function and blood clotting. Milk and other dairy foods such as yogurt and most cheeses are the best sources of calcium. In addition, dark green leafy vegetables, fish with edible bones, and calcium-fortified foods supply significant amounts.

carotenoids Derived from the antioxidant vitamin A, these yellow, orange, and red pigments are synthesized by plants. The most common carotenoids are alpha-carotene, beta-carotene, beta-cryptoxanthin, lutein, lycopene, and zeaxanthin.

catechins A type of flavonoid found in tea, catechins provide the health benefits of neutralizing free radicals and possibly reducing the risk of cancer.

cholesterol A waxy, fatlike substance that occurs naturally in all parts of the body. Your body needs some cholesterol to work properly. But high levels of cholesterol in the blood can block arteries and increase the risk of heart disease.

choline Although the body manufactures some of this essential nutrient linked to heart health and cancer prevention, we need dietary sources, too; beef and eggs are good sources.

coenzyme Q10 A fat-soluble compound primarily synthesized by the body and also consumed in the diet, coenzyme Q10 acts as an antioxidant in cell membranes. Food sources include nuts, herring, trout, and soybean and canola oils.

coronary artery disease (CAD) The most common type of heart disease, coronary artery disease is the leading cause of death in the United States for both men and women. The arteries that supply blood to the heart muscle become hardened and narrowed due to the buildup of cholesterol and other material, called plaque, on their inner walls. As the buildup grows, less blood can flow through the arteries. As a result, the heart muscle can't get the blood or oxygen it needs. This can lead to chest pain (angina) or a heart attack.

cortisol A stress hormone manufactured by the adrenal and pituitary glands.

curcumin A polyphenolic compound that gives turmeric its yellow color, and an antioxidant that may be linked to cognitive function.

DHA An omega-3 fatty acid, docosahexaenoic acid (DHA) is essential for the growth and functional development of the brain in infants and for maintenance of normal brain function in adults.

diallyl sulfide A type of sulfide found in onions, garlic, olives, leeks, and scallions, diallyl sulfide may provide the health benefits of lowering LDL cholesterol and maintaining a healthy immune system.

EGCG Epigallocatechin-3-gallate (EGCG) is a type of catechin found in green tea. It has been linked to heart health, lower cancer risks, and weight loss.

ellagic acid A natural cancer-fighting agent found in strawberries.

essential fatty acids Alpha-linolenic acid (ALA), an omega-3 fatty acid, and linoleic acid (LA), an omega-6 fatty acid, are considered essential fatty acids because they cannot be synthesized by humans.

ferulic acid A type of phenol found in various fruits and vegetables and citrus fruits, ferulic acid has antioxidant-like activities that may reduce the risk of degenerative diseases, heart disease, and eye disease.

flavanols A type of flavonoid found in citrus fruits, which provides the health benefits of neutralizing free radicals and possibly reducing the risk of cancer.

flavones A type of flavonoid that includes apigenin and luteolin, found in parsley, thyme, celery, and hot peppers.

flavonoids A subgroup of polyphenols, flavonoids are naturally occurring compounds found in plant-based foods recognized as conferring certain health benefits. So far, there are more than 4,000 known flavonoid compounds, including anthocyanidins; flavanones, including catechins, found in teas (particularly green and white), chocolate, grapes, berries, and apples; theaflavins and thearubigins, found in teas (particularly black and oolong); and proanthocyanidins, found in chocolate, apples, berries, red grapes, and red wine. The flavonoid category also includes the widely distributed quercetin, kaempferol, myricetin, and isorhamnetin, which are found in yellow onions, scallions, kale, broccoli, apples, berries, and teas.

folic acid A B vitamin, this helps the body make healthy new cells. Folic acid is critical for pregnant women, to prevent major birth defects in the baby's brain or spine. Food sources include leafy green vegetables, fruits, dried beans, peas, and nuts. Enriched breads, cereals, and other grain products also contain folic acid.

free radicals Highly reactive substances that result from exposure to oxygen, background radiation, and other environmental factors. Free radicals cause cellular damage in the body. The damage may be repaired by antioxidants.

HDL cholesterol High-density lipoprotein, or HDL, is known as the good, or "happy," cholesterol, which carries about one-fourth to one-third of blood cholesterol. High levels of HDL seem to protect against heart attack. Low levels of HDL (less than 40 milligrams per deciliter) increase the risk of heart disease. Medical experts think that HDL tends to carry cholesterol away from the arteries and back to the liver, where it's passed from the body. Some experts believe that HDL removes excess cholesterol from arterial plaque, slowing its buildup.

hydrogenated fat During food processing, fats may undergo a chemical process called hydrogenation. This is common in margarine and shortening. Hydrogenated fats raise blood cholesterol levels.

isoflavones Another subclass of flavonoids, these include daidzein, genistein, and glycitein and are found in soybeans, soy foods, and legumes.

L-carnitine A derivative of the amino acid lysine. Healthy individuals manufacture enough of this substance, which plays an important role in cellular activity, converting long chain fatty acids so the body can use them.

LDL cholesterol Also known as the bad, or "lousy," cholesterol, low-density cholesterol can slowly build up in the inner walls of the arteries that feed the heart and brain. Together with other substances, it can form plaque, a thick, hard deposit that can narrow the arteries and make them less flexible. This condition is known as atherosclerosis. If a clot forms and blocks a narrowed artery, a heart attack or stroke can result.

L-ergothioneine A powerful antioxidant linked to heart health and found in mushrooms.

lignans Lignan precursors are found in a wide variety of plant-based foods, including seeds, whole grains, legumes, fruits, and vegetables; when they are eaten, they are converted to the mammalian lignans, enterodiol and enterolactone, by bacteria that normally colonize the human intestine. Flaxseeds are the richest dietary source of lignan precursors.

lipoic acid Alpha-lipoic acid (LA), also known as thioctic acid, is a naturally occurring compound that is synthesized in small amounts by humans and is found in some foods. Although it is an antioxidant itself, lipoic acid also regenerates other antioxidants after they've been oxidized by their scavenging activity.

lutein A carotenoid, this antioxidant is best known for its association with healthy eyes. Lutein is abundant in green, leafy vegetables such as collard greens, spinach, and kale.

lycopene A carotenoid, this potent antioxidant is found in tomatoes, watermelon, guavas, papayas, apricots, pink grapefruit, blood oranges, and other foods. Estimates suggest 85 percent of American dietary intake of lycopene comes from tomatoes and tomato products.

minerals The body uses minerals for many different jobs, including building bones, making hormones, and regulating heartbeat. There are two kinds: Your body needs *macrominerals* in larger amounts, and these include calcium, chloride, magnesium, phosphorus, potassium, sodium, and sulfur. Your body needs just small amounts of *trace minerals*. These include cobalt, copper, fluoride, iodine, iron, manganese, selenium, and zinc.

omega-3 fatty acids A type of fatty acid found in fish and marine oils, omega-3s provide the health benefits of reduced risk of cardiovascular disease and improved mental and visual function.

oxidation The loss of electrons from a compound (or element) in a chemical reaction. When one compound is oxidized, another compound is reduced. That is, the other compound must "pick up" the electrons that the first has lost.

oxytocin An octapeptide hormone secreted by the pituitary gland, it stimulates the contraction of uterine muscle and the secretion of milk; production is stimulated by orgasm and cuddling. Oxytocin is linked to lower rates of breast cancer and has some antioxidant properties.

pectin A natural gelling agent found in ripe fruit, pectin is an important source of fiber.

phenol See polyphenols.

phytochemicals (also called phytonutrients) Technically, these are any chemicals produced by plants, but the term is generally used to describe compounds that may affect health but are not essential nutrients.

phytosterols Plant-derived compounds that are similar in structure and function to cholesterol.

polyphenols Researchers say these are the most abundant dietary antioxidants, and the main sources are fruits and plant-derived beverages, such as juices, tea, coffee, and red wine. Polyphenols are made up of phenols, a class of chemical compounds consisting of a hydroxyl functional group.

resveratrol A polyphenolic compound linked to heart health and found in grapes, red wine, purple grape juice, peanuts, and some berries.

retinoids Derivatives of vitamin A, retinoids are topical and oral antioxidants that are used to prevent and reverse sun damage and signs of aging, as well as to treat acne. These medications should be prescribed and coordinated by a qualified licensed health care professional. Vitamin A supplements should not be used in tandem with these drugs due to a risk of increased toxicity.

saponins The functional component of soybeans, soy foods, and soy protein, saponins may lower LDL cholesterol and may contain anticancer enzymes.

saturated fat The main dietary cause of high blood cholesterol, found mostly in foods from animals and some plants, including beef, beef fat, veal, lamb, pork, lard, poultry fat, butter, cream, milk, cheeses, and other dairy products made from whole and 2 percent milk. All of these foods also contain dietary cholesterol. Foods from plants that contain saturated fat include coconut, coconut oil, palm oil, and palm kernel oil (often called tropical oils), and cocoa butter.

selenium While this is a mineral, not an antioxidant nutrient, it is a component of antioxidant enzymes. Plant foods such as rice and wheat are the major dietary sources of selenium in most countries. The amount of selenium in soil, which varies by region, determines the amount of selenium in the foods grown in that soil. Animals that eat grains or plants grown in selenium-rich soil have higher levels of selenium in their muscle. Meats, bread, and Brazil nuts are good food sources.

serotonin A hormone manufactured by the brain, serotonin is a feel-good chemical that, along with dopamine, has been shown to have antioxidant properties.

soluble fiber A type of dietary fiber found in psyllium, cereals, oatmeal, apples, citrus fruits, beans, and other foods, which increases the viscosity in the gut and acts to reduce high blood cholesterol levels.

superoxide dismutase enzyme An antioxidant enzyme produced in the body.

trans fatty acids Found in small amounts in various animal products such as beef, pork, and lamb and in the butterfat in butter and milk, trans fatty acids are also formed during the process of hydrogenation, making margarine, shortening, cooking oils, and the foods made from them a major source of trans fats in the American diet. Partially hydrogenated vegetable oils provide about three-fourths of the trans fats in the US diet. Trans fatty acids are also formed during the process of hydrogenation.

triglycerides A form of fat made in the body. Elevated triglycerides can be due to overweight/obesity, physical inactivity, cigarette smoking, excess alcohol consumption, or a diet very high in carbohydrates (60 percent of total calories or more). People with high triglycerides often have a high total cholesterol level, including a high LDL (bad) level and a low HDL (good) level. Many people with heart disease and/or diabetes also have high triglyceride levels.

unsaturated fats Polyunsaturated and monounsaturated fats are the two unsaturated fats. They're found mainly in many fish, nuts, seeds, and oils from plants. Some examples of foods that contain these fats include salmon, trout, herring, avocados, olives, walnuts, and liquid vegetable oils such as soybean, corn, safflower, canola, olive, and sunflower. Both polyunsaturated and monounsaturated fats may help lower your blood cholesterol level when you use them in place of saturated and trans fats.

vitamin One of many organic compounds that are nutritionally essential in small amounts to control metabolic processes and cannot be synthesized by the body. Vitamins are usually classified by their solubility, which to some degree determines their stability; occurrence in foodstuffs; distribution in body fluids; and tissue storage capacity. While there are many vitamins, vitamins A, C, and E have the strongest antioxidant properties.

vitamin A Also known as retinol (because it produces the pigments in the retina of the eye) and carotenoids, this is a fat-soluble antioxidant vitamin. It helps form and maintain healthy teeth, skeletal and soft tissue, mucous membranes, and skin. Retinol is an active form of vitamin A found in animal liver, whole milk, and some fortified foods.

vitamin C See ascorbic acid.

vitamin E Also known as alpha-tocopherol, this antioxidant is found in almonds; in many oils, including wheat germ, safflower, corn, and soybean oils; and in mangoes, nuts, broccoli, and other foods. It's also important in the formation of red blood cells and helps the body use vitamin K.

xanthone An antioxidant found in the tropical fruit mangosteen.

zeaxanthin A type of carotenoid, found in eggs, citrus fruits, and corn, that contributes to the maintenance of eyesight.

Endnotes

Chapter 1

[1] Judy McBride, "High-ORAC Foods May Slow Aging," Agricultural Research Service, February 8, 1999.

[2] Do-Hoon Kim, Yoo-Sun Moon, Hee-Sung Kim, Jun-Sub Jung, Hyung-Moo Park, Hong-Won Suh, Yung-Hi Kim, and Dong-Keun Song, "Effect of Zen Meditation on Serum Nitric Oxide Activity and Lipid Peroxidation," *Progress in Neuro-Psychopharmacology and Biological Psychiatry* 29, no. 2 (February 2005): 327–31.

[3] L. Hallberg, L. Hulthén, C. Bengtsson, L. Lapidus, and G. Lindstedt, "Iron Balance in Menstruating Women," *European Journal of Clinical Nutrition* 49, no. 3 (March 1995): 200–207.

Chapter 2

[1] "Almonds May Help in Weight Loss; Almond Diet Sheds More Pounds Than Low-Fat, High-Carb Diet," WebMD Health News, November 7, 2003, www.webmd.com/diet/news/20031107/almonds-may-help-in-weight-loss.

[2] Alan Mozes, "Antioxidant-Rich Foods Lose Nutritional Luster Over Time," Medicinenet.com, April 2, 2009, www.medicinenet.com/script/main/art.asp?articlekey=99057.

[3] "Grapefruit and Weight Loss," Medicalnewstoday.com, January 24, 2004, www.medicalnewstoday.com/articles/5495.php.

[4] Michael B. Zemel, Warren Thompson, Anita Milstead, Kristin Morris, and Peter Campbell, "Dietary Calcium and Dairy Acceleration of Weight and Fat Loss during Energy Restriction in Obese Adults," *Obesity Research* 12, no. 4 (2004): 582–90, www.nature.com/oby/journal/v12/n4/full/oby200467a.html.

[5] Joe A. Vinson, Ligia Zubik, Pratima Bose, Najwa Samman, and John Proch, "Dried Fruits: Excellent in Vitro and in Vivo Antioxidants," *Journal of the American College of Nutrition* 24, no. 1 (2005): 44–50, www.jacn.org/cgi/content/abstract/24/1/44.

[6] Martha Filipic, "Study: Fats in Avocados Help Body Absorb Carotenoids," Ohio State University News Service, March 15, 2005, http://extension.osu.edu/~news/story.php?id=3065.

[7] Sui, Xuemei, MD; Michael J. LaMonte, PhD; James N. Laditka, PhD; James W. Hardin, PhD; Nancy Chase, BS; Steven P. Hooker, PhD; Steven N. Blair, PED; "Cardiorespiratory Fitness and Adiposity as Mortality Predictors in Older Adults," *The Journal of the American Medical Association* 298, no. 21 (December 5, 2007): 2507–2516.

[8] Shirin Hooshmand and Bahram H. Arjmandi, "Viewpoint: Dried Plum, an Emerging Functional Food That May Effectively Improve Bone Health," *Ageing Research Reviews* 8, no. 2 (April 2009): 122–27.

[9] "Tart Cherries May Reduce Factors Associated with Heart Disease and Diabetes," University of Michigan Health Services Newsroom, April 7, 2009, www2.med.umich.edu/prmc/media/newsroom/details.cfm?ID=148.

[10] Diet and Lifestyle Recommendations, American Heart Association, http://heart.org/presenter.jhtml?identifier=851.

[11] Rosalie Marion Bliss, "Study Shows Consuming Hibiscus Tea Lowers Blood Pressure," Agricultural Research Service, www.ars.usda.gov/is/pr/2008/081110.htm.

[12] Ella Haddad, Pera Jambazian, Martina Karunia, Jay Tanzman, and Joan Sabaté, "A Pecan-Enriched Diet Increases Y-tocopherol/cholesterol and Decreases Thiobarbituric Acid Reactive Substances in Plasma of Adults," *Nutrition Research* 26, no. 8: 397–402.

[13] A. Venket Rao and Sanjiv Agarwal, "Role of Antioxidant Lycopene in Cancer and Heart Disease," *Journal of the American College of Nutrition* 19, no. 5 (2000): 563–69, www.jacn.org/cgi/content/full/19/5/563.

[14] Miranda Hitti, "Traffic Stress? Cinnamon, Peppermint May Help," WebMD Health News, April 28, 2005, www.webmd.com/food-recipes/news/20050428/traffic-stress-cinnamon-peppermint-may-help.

[15] "Spinach, Broccoli May Help Keep the Brain Young," Fisher Center for Alzheimer's Research Foundation, July 20, 2004, www.alzinfo.org/newsarticle/templates/archivenewstemplate.asp?articleid=109&zoneid=9.

[16] "Breakfast Practices and Cognitive and Academic Performance in Children," Breakfast Research Institute, May 3, 2007, www.breakfastresearchinstitute.org/breakfastsciencelibrary/viewarticle.cfm?articleID=866.

[17] "Diet for Stress Management: Stress-Reducing Foods," Medicinenet.com, www.medicinenet.com/diet_for_stress_management_pictures_slideshow/article.htm.

[18] "Weekly Curry 'May Fight Dementia,'" BBC News, June 3, 2009, http://news.bbc.co.uk/2/hi/health/8080630.stm.

Chapter 3

[1] "Obesity among U.S. Adults Continues to Rise," Centers for Disease Control and Prevention press release, July 8, 2009, www.cdc.gov/media/pressrel/2009/r090708.htm.

[2] "New Obesity Survey: Many Americans Think They're 'Lighter' Than They Are, Most *Not* Being Told by a Doctor They Need to Lose Weight," National Consumers League press release, June 19, 2007, www.nclnet.org/news/2007/obesity_survey_06192007.htm.

[3] G. Schulze, "Sleep Protects Excitatory Cortical Circuits against Oxidative Damage," *Medical Hypotheses* 63, no. 2 (2004): 203–7.

[4] William Dement, "Sleepless at Stanford," www.stanford.edu/~dement/sleepless.html.

[5] Carol A. Everson, Christa D. Laatsch, and Neil Hogg, "Antioxidant Defense Responses to Sleep Loss and Sleep Recovery," *American Journal of Physiology—Regulatory, Integrative, and Comparative Physiology* 288, no. 2 (February 2005): R374–R383.

[6] William L. Haskell, Steven N. Blair, and James O. Hill, "Physical Activity: Health Outcomes and Importance for Public Health Policy," *Preventive Medicine*, May 2009.

[7] Summary, "Physical Activity and Health: A Report of the Surgeon General," Centers for Disease Control and Prevention, www.cdc.gov/NCCDPHP/SGR/summ.htm.

[8] Claudia Di Giacomo, Rosaria Acquaviva, Valeria Sorrenti, Angelo Vanella, Salvatore Grasso, Maria Luisa Barcellona, Fabio Galvano, Luca Vanella, and Marcella Renis, "Oxidative and Antioxidant Status in Plasma of Runners: Effect of Oral Supplementation with Natural Antioxidants," *Journal of Medicinal Food* 12, no. 1 (February 2009): 145–50.

[9] Martin J. Gibala and Sean L. McGee, "Metabolic Adaptations to Short-Term High-Intensity Interval Training: A Little Pain for a Lot of Gain?" *Exercise and Sport Sciences Reviews* 36, no. 2 (April 2008): 58–63.

[10] John A. Babraj, Niels B. J. Vollaard, Cameron Keast, Fergus M. Guppy, Greg Cottrell, and James A. Timmons, "Extremely Short Duration High Intensity Interval Training Substantially Improves Insulin Action in Young Healthy Males," *BMC Endocrine Disorders* 9, no. 3 (2009), doi:10.1186/1472-6823-9-3.

[11] N. Hattori et al., "Changes of ROS during a Two-Day Ultra-marathon Race," *International Journal of Sports Medicine* 30, no. 6 (June 2009): 426–29, Epub 2009 Feb 6.

[12] Bente Klarlund Pedersen and Laurie Hoffman-Goetz, "Exercise and the Immune System: Regulation, Integration, and Adaptation," *Physiological Reviews* 80, no. 3 (July 2000): 1,055–81, http://physrev.physiology.org/cgi/content/full/80/3/1055.

[13] "Can Exercise Reduce Your Risk of Catching a Cold?" American Council on Exercise, www.acefitness.org/fitfacts/fitfacts_display.aspx?itemid=2613.

[14] Marc Berman, John Jonides, and Stephen Kaplan, "The Cognitive Benefits of Interacting with Nature," *Psychological Science* 19, no. 12 (December 2008): 1,207–12(6).

[15] Rick Weiss, "Noise Pollution Takes Toll on Health and Happiness," *Washington Post,* June 5, 2007, page HE05, www.washingtonpost.com/wp-dyn/content/article/2007/06/04/AR2007060401430.html.

[16] B. C. Wolverton, "Foliage Plants for Improving Indoor Air Quality," NASA Technical Reports, presented at the National Foliage Foundation Interiorscape Seminar, Hollywood, FL, July 19, 1988.

[17] "Antioxidants Fight Smog Damage," BBC News, September 9, 2001, http://news.bbc.co.uk/2/hi/health/1552074.stm.

[18] Bob Berkowitz and Susan Yager-Berkowitz, "Expert Advice: Withholding Sex," thirdage.com, www.thirdage.com/sex/expert-advice-withholding-sex.

[19] R. L. Kolotkin, M. Binks, R. D. Crosby, T. Østbye, R. E. Gress, and T. D. Abrams, "Obesity and Sexual Quality of Life," *Obesity* 14, no. 3 (March 2006): 472–79.

[20] S. Amaral, P. J. Oliveira, and J. Ramahlo-Santos, "Diabetes and the Impairment of Reproductive Function: Possible Role of Mitochondria and Reactive Oxygen Species," *Current Diabetes Review* 4, no. 1 (February 2008): 46–54, www.ncbi.nlm.nih.gov/pubmed/18220695.

[21] Colette Bouchez, "Better Sex: What's Weight Got to Do with It?" WebMD.com, March 25, 2005, www.webmd.com/sex-relationships/guide/sex-and-weight.

[22] Karen M. Grewen, Susan S. Girdler, Janet Amico, and Kathleen C. Light, "Effects of Partner Support on Resting Oxytocin, Cortisol, Norepinephrine, and Blood Pressure before and after Warm Partner Contact," *Psychosomatic Medicine* 67 (2005): 531–38.

[23] Claudia Camerino, "Low Sympathetic Tone and Obese Phenotype in Oxytocin-Deficient Mice," *Obesity* 17, no. 5 (2009): 980–84, doi:10.1038/oby.2009.12, www.nature.com/oby/journal/v17/n5/abs/oby200912a.html.

[24] Karen M. Grewen, Susan S. Girdler, Janet Amico, and Kathleen C. Light, "Effects of Partner Support on Resting Oxytocin, Cortisol, Norepinephrine, and Blood Pressure before and after Warm Partner Contact," *Psychosomatic Medicine* 67 (2005): 531–38.

[25] Roni Caryn Rabin, "Breast-Feeding Benefits Mothers, Study Finds," *New York Times,* April 21, 2009, www.nytimes.com/2009/04/22/health/research/22breast.html.

[26] J. C. Kefer, S. Agarwal, and E. Sabanegh, "Role of Antioxidants in the Treatment of Male Infertility," *International Journal of Urology* 16, no. 5 (May 2009): 449–57, Epub 2009 Apr 6.

[27] S. S. Mehendale, A. S. Kilari Bams, C. S. Deshmukh, B. S. Dhorepatil, V. N. Nimbargi, and S. R. Joshi, "Oxidative Stress-Mediated Essential Polyunsaturated Fatty Acid Alterations in Female Infertility," *Human Fertility* 12, no. 1 (March 2009): 28–33.

[28] "Soy and Flax Are Natural Alternatives to Hormone Replacement Therapy," *Friedman Nutrition Notes,* September 2002, http://nutrition.tufts.edu/docs/NutritionNotes/2002-09.html.

Chapter 6

[1] "Thirty-One Percent of Americans Never Use Sunscreen," *Consumer Reports* press release, May 20, 2009, http://pressroom.consumerreports.org/pressroom/2009/05/consumer-reports-poll-thirty-one-percent-of-americans-never-use-sunscreen.html.

[2] Judy R. Rees, Therese A. Stukel, Ann E. Perry, Michael S. Zens, Steven K. Spencer, and Margaret R. Karagas, "Tea Consumption and Basal Cell and Squamous Cell Skin Cancer: Results of a Case Control Study," *Journal of the American Academy of Dermatology* 56, no. 5 (May 2007): 781–85.

Chapter 7

[1] Patrick J. McDonnell, "Acai Has Gone from Staple of the Amazon to Global Wonder-Berry," *Los Angeles Times,* September 21, 2008, www.latimes.com/news/nationworld/world/latinamerica/la-fg-acai21-2008sep21,0,2627228.story?track=rs.

[2] Liz Applegate, "Yes, You Can: Canned Foods Are Healthier and Tastier Than You Might Think," *Runner's World,* December 29, 2003, www.runnersworld.com/article/0,7120,s6-242-300--6028-0,00.html.

[3] Jennifer A. Nettleton, Pamela L. Lutsey, Youfa Wang, João A. Lima, Erin D. Michos, and David R. Jacobs Jr., "Diet Soda Intake and Risk of Incident Metabolic Syndrome and Type 2 Diabetes in the Multi-Ethnic Study of Atherosclerosis (MESA)," *Diabetes Care* 32, no. 4 (April 2009): 688–94, Epub 2009 Jan 16.

Acknowledgments

There are so many people who make my life better each day that it would be impossible to list each and every one of you! I will try to name a few.

First, thank you to my clients, who truly are the root of everything I do. There is no greater joy than to learn from you, watch you grow, and see you succeed. Thank you for giving me the experience and motivation to write this book.

I would not be able to write this book if it were not for all of the outstanding women in my nutrition practice. Thank you Lilly Cannold for your hard work and dedication. Thank you to the associates, Lara Metz, Amanda Buthmann, and Daria Ventura. Your clients are lucky and so am I. Lara, I am forever grateful for your commitment to the practice and passion for what we do, for your tremendous heart and good sense, and most of all for your friendship. To the interns who helped in so many ways on this book—Alexandra Kaplan, Deborah Tagliareni, Lauren Deutsch, Lauren Rosen, Brigitte Zeitlin—thank you for your enthusiasm for this project.

This book truly would not have come to life without my absolutely brilliant writing partner, Sarah Mahoney. You are not only a fabulous writer, but you are also a friend, a true joy to work with, and you kept me sane throughout this process. Thank you, Sarah!

Thank you to my recipe developer, Therese Baran. You understood my love of antioxidant-rich food from day one and made life more delicious.

I can't give a big enough THANK YOU to everyone at Rodale books who had a vision for this book from the start! Thank you to Karen Rinaldi, Nancy N. Bailey, Fran Minerva, Jessica Lee, Yelena Gitlin, Beth Tarson, and Chris Rhoads. Finally, Shannon Welch, thank you for being the hardest-working, most-creative, on-top-of it editor I could ask for. You're a pleasure to work with and I thank you from the bottom of my heart for all of your enthusiasm! Thank you to the talented and brilliant experts who shared their love of antioxidants in Chapter 5!

Thank you everyone at William Morris Endeavor . . . especially Mel Berger, for opening my eyes to the cornerstone of this book and truly bringing it to life. Thank you Ken Slotnick for your never-ending energy and support of everything I do. Thank you Strand Conover, Jeff Googel, Andy Muser, and Bethany Dick for your hard work. Thank you Ben Simone, Suzanne Lyon, Graham Jaenicke, and Miles Gidaly for all of your hard work.

Thank you to everyone at CBS's *The Early Show,* especially Susie Shackman, Dina Blau, and Betsy Alexander for your continued support!

To everyone at *Women's Health* magazine—Michele Promaulayko, Jill Waldbieser, Allison Keane, Erin Clinton, and the rest of the incredible team. It is an honor to be part of your family. I am grateful for the opportunity to work with such smart, talented, and fun people.

I feel blessed every day for my truly amazing friends. Thank you for being the "emergency contacts" for my kids *and* for me! You have all lent your ears, offered amazing words of wisdom, and brought so much fun, laughter, and love into my life.

How could I possibly thank you enough, Mom and Dad? You always encouraged me to "go for it" in life and gave me the courage to always follow my dreams and take chances. I am so blessed to have you for parents.

Thank you, Judd and Samantha Karofsky, for your friendship; Judd, you tortured me through childhood but I would not get through adulthood without you and your unwavering support.

To my little man, Rex, thank you for your genuine interest in whether "broccoli has protein," for being so open to trying new foods, and for your morning hugs and kisses. To my little bean, Maizy, thank you for all of your "Mommy I love you SO much" squeezes. You both make my heart skip a beat daily and are truly the O_2 of my life.

Finally, to my husband, Brett, for making sure I keep everything in perspective every day, and for truly understanding my passion.

Index

Boldface page references indicate illustrations. Underscored references indicate boxed text.

About the Author

Keri Glassman, MS, RD, CDN, has a thriving nutrition practice in New York City and helps millions as a contributing editor to *Women's Health* magazine. She counsels individuals on a broad range of challenges—from weight loss to improving energy. A distinguished expert in the field of nutrition, she has appeared on the *Today* show, *Good Morning America*, *The View*, *The Doctors,* and *Dr. Oz*. Glassman holds a masters of science degree in clinical nutrition from New York University. She was an All-American lacrosse player at Tufts University and has completed the New York City Marathon and several triathlons. She resides in Manhattan with her husband, Brett, and their children, Rex and Maizy.

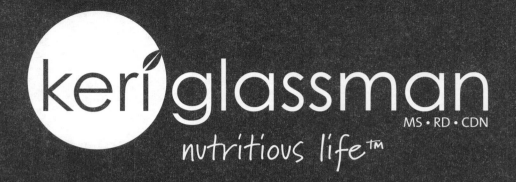

keri glassman
MS · RD · CDN

nutritious life™

Keri is passionate about customizing your perfect diet and helping you achieve a nutritious life.

For an online monthly membership, which includes more recipes, support, and meal plans, log on to: **WWW.THEO2DIET.COM**

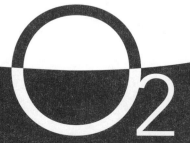